IGNITING
RESILIENCE

IGNITING RESILIENCE

Overcoming the Despair of Receiving a Death Sentence

By

CHRISTINE BURNS

With Dr Elizabeth Pritchard

DISCLAIMER

All the information, techniques and concepts contained within this publication are of the nature of general comment only and are not in any way recommended as individual advice. The intent is to offer a variety of information to provide a wider range of choices now and in the future, recognising that we all have widely diverse circumstances and viewpoints.
I would like to honour my own journey and those of other inspiring researchers and authors who I've had the privilege of studying and who are credited in this book. Thank you for supporting me in finding the courage to voice my discoveries. Should any reader choose to make use of the information contained herein, this is their decision, and the contributors (and their companies), authors and publishers do not assume any responsibilities whatsoever under any condition or circumstances. It is recommended that the reader obtain their own independent advice.

First Edition, Published 2022
by Christine Burns

ISBN 978-0-6455380-0-7 (Softcover)
ISBN 978-0-6455380-1-4 (Epub)
ISBN 978-0-6455380-3-8 (Kindle)
ISBN 978-0-6455380-2-1 (Audio)

Author: Christine Burns
Igniting Resilience: Overcoming the Despair of Receiving
a Death Sentence / Christine Burns

To Mum and Dad (Janet and Bill Burns)
You taught me what it is to be courageous, curious and most
of all, how to have fun no matter what life throws our way.
And yes, Mum you are right 'there is always a way'!

TABLE OF CONTENTS

SECTION FOUR: PURPOSEFUL INTENTION

SECTION FIVE: THE EMPOWERMENT

INTRODUCTION

On the morning of 2nd November, 2016, I answered the phone like I had any other time, "hello Christine speaking". It was one of my surgeons who had operated on me for an emergency hysterectomy the week before. They said they would ring the following week and check up to see how I was going with recovery.

After the pleasantries were exchanged, the next words I heard were, "You have endometrial cancer". I was totally floored, speechless, and not sure of what to say or do next. I managed to voice some expletives, but that was about it.

From that moment on my life changed, completely. I found myself going from oncology waiting rooms to cancer treatment rooms. Injected with radioactive dye and forced to lie completely still for an hour while it worked its way through my system, to give the medical staff a better image of what was going on. Tattooed for treatment. Asked invasive questions, and revealing whatever it took so I could get to the next step of treatment, and then recovery.

I was also asking myself a whole lot of questions. Why did this have to happen to me? I'm fit and healthy and take care of myself. Why? It turns out these waiting and treatment rooms provided me with the opportunity to interrogate every part of my own life and were not just a way to make sense of tragedy.

Just two weeks before, I was writing exams, delivering lectures, teaching tutorials and providing pastoral care for tertiary students as they neared the end of another academic year. I was in full swing, working long hours to make sure the students could give their best at this time of year. I was active, working out, riding my bike, contributing to society, participating as an equal in a married relationship. I was having fun.

In the midst of this gut-wrenching turmoil when I thought my life was about to end sooner than I had ever anticipated, I had a brief moment of clarity. I pledged to myself that I would do everything I possibly could to look after me – mentally, physically and emotionally. The medical crew could do their thing, and together we would tackle this cancer as a strong united team. I knew if we combined our strengths, we would have the best shot at achieving success.

No matter what obstacles I had come up against in the past, I had always progressed through those times with a strong team unit around me. The best times in my life, sport and work, were when we all had each other's backs. We would do whatever was needed for each other to be the best versions of ourselves and achieve success.

And the opposite was true. The toughest times were when there was no concept of 'team'. Instead there was a competitive environment with people who had no idea how to bring out the best in each other, how to work together, or how to accomplish the end goal.

The diagnosis was a definite wakeup call. On the outside I looked like I had everything together. I had graduated from university, good job, recently married, living in a big city, doing well, enjoying life, and so far had achieved a great deal. But on the inside I was conflicted, as at 44, I hadn't yet done the things I wanted to do in life.

I was not ready to let go of who I was or who I wanted to become. I was scared and not ready to die! I still wanted to contribute to people in a way that could change their lives and assist them to be the best versions of themselves. I wanted to be successful, rebel against the status quo, and leave a legacy that would inspire others to achieve anything they wanted to.

My wise Scottish Mum frequently said to me, "There is always a way. If you really want something and are committed to it with all your might, then you can achieve whatever you want". As a youngster I would ride around on my bicycle with a feeling of pure happiness. I had fun riding effortlessly over jumps, and doing skids as if nothing in the world could ever go wrong. And when it did go wrong and I fell off, I would hear my Mum telling me to get back up on my bike and carry on.

When I played indoor hockey for New Zealand as a goalkeeper, I would defend the goal with the utmost determination and focus. I would give my absolute best in my role, no matter how intense or close the game was, no matter what abuse was hurled at me. I steadfastly maintained our team objective.

These were some of the lessons I knew best: to always have fun and cultivate a feeling of happiness (optimism); to get back up and go again no matter what; and to give my absolute best to the team because a team works best when we have each other's back.

These lessons were the ones I needed to engage at the time of being diagnosed - to help me get through the life-threatening challenges and the unknowns of what was to come. Progressing through childhood into adulthood with parents who instilled these lessons into everything I did and thought, helped me develop a robust level of resilience.

Resilience is that ability to adapt, to overcome, to work through the challenges in life and go on again with an optimistic view. In the moment of that phone call, I had to decide whether to call on every ounce of resilience I had built up so far, or fall off my bike for the last time and not get back up.

Whether it was a setback at school, sport, work, or life in general, I was encouraged to identify possible solutions to cope and deal with uncontrollable moments. When fear raised its head, I was taught that it's better to face it than run from it, and who knows there might actually be some fun to be had. At the very least there was always an opportunity to learn something new.

When Mum used to say, "Oh well the sun will still shine tomorrow", she meant there will always be a new day and a new way to work things out. So keep going and do not give up. I took from this that if I could just keep moving forward and take back my power little by little, there would always be a way.

When it gets really tough, we need to be thankful and grateful for who and what we have around us. Recognise the moments of joy, the times of laughter, and be totally in the moment, because it's all we truly have. It was in these moments that I could fill up my own 'tank' to gain some strength and energy.

Dad used to say, "If you are going to do something, make a good job of it". I believed he was referring to both the good and the tough times. So here I was, knowing that to get through these horrendous moments and whatever the future had in store for me, I had to make a good job of it, because I might only get one shot.

I chose to get up, get on with it, and give it my all. I combined my strengths with the greatest team I could possibly muster around me. Together as a strong cohesive team we would be formidable. Now was the time for action. It was a time for 'less chit chat and more do'. It was a time to hunker down and give it all I had. I needed to combine not only my brawn and determination, but my brains as well. Even when I was scared or worried, I had to just go ahead and take action. I had to ask for help and I had to be vulnerable. This was not something I could do on my own.

Having an academic background and being a closet geek, I knew there would be many pieces of research I could draw on to help me create

CHRISTINE BURNS

my best environment, mindset, physiology, and provide a way forward during this time. I invested in research from the areas of positive and performance psychology, the science of happiness and subjective well-being, the old life lessons from Greek philosophers, and the sciences of physiology, biology and exercise. Together, these philosophies and truths paved the path for me to rise above the diagnosis, not accept the prognosis, and thrive in every area of my life.

This book is designed to help you achieve this as well. You do not necessarily need a diagnosis – it could be adversity in any shape or form. The principles I share in this book will assist you to cultivate the best possible game plan and then take action with determination and focus. It is also important to have fun while doing it. To engage the laughter in the lighter side of the moments whenever you can.

When setbacks, trauma, adversity or challenges appear, we can make the conscious decision to get caught up in the negativity of it, give away our power and succumb to the harshness of the situation, or we can face our fear, make friends with the moment, and activate our resilience superpower. I will explain how.

This book is about the lessons I've learned, the knowledge I've gained, and my efforts to embody these in everyday life. This ensured that I would thrive and not just survive, while discovering the limitless possibilities within this journey of adversity.

You can too!

The Diagnosis

* * *

Affirmation: "I allow myself to feel the emotion"

Chapter 1

Uncontrollable Moments

O n that fateful November morning at 11:19 a.m. I answered a phone call that changed my life forever! My surgeon, Carmel, rang one week after major surgery and said, "We've got the pathology results back and I need to tell you that you have endometrial cancer".

Time appeared to stop. There was no noise, nothing. The only sensation I had at that moment was a slow tightening across my chest. My thoughts spun in all directions, with many different internal conversations occurring simultaneously. I gradually came back to the present moment, with my surgeon still on the phone, and had what I call a *nano tanty*. This consisted of a number of profanities spilling forth, along with a massive surge of adrenaline throughout my body.

I realised I had stopped breathing for a moment. As I began to breathe again, I knew I needed to turn my ears on and listen carefully. The main thought running through my head was to shut up and listen, and get on top of my emotions. I knew I had to tune in and be the best version of myself in this situation.

I felt my senses go from being aware of everything, and then in an instant, to only hearing and feeling Carmel's voice through my earphones. I finely tuned into each word she spoke so I could hear all the details. I heard the word *treatable* and that got me into 'game on' mode. That was all I needed to hear. "It is treatable".

Thoughts raced quickly through my head. "I am on a call from my surgeon. She has just given me shocking news. I don't know what all this means. What is the first thing I need to do?" After the initial shock of hearing the words "you have endometrial cancer", I began thinking, "Okay, you guys do your bit medically and I will do the rest mentally, physically and emotionally". If I was allotted to *this game* now, then I would play it at my best.

The phone call ended. I went outside into our garden and sat there in shock. I was thinking, "What the hell just happened? How could this happen to me? What have I done to deserve this? Who's playing a joke on me?" Then it started to sink in, just a little. My life had just changed… forever! This *thing*, the news of my diagnosis, was out of my control and now it was up to me to decide on a response. What that response would be I wasn't quite sure, but deep down I knew I would find one.

I walked in and out of the house thinking, "What the hell? This wasn't in my life plan". I was only 44. I was recovering remarkably well post-emergency hysterectomy and then this had to happen!

I sat there with tears in my eyes, biting my bottom lip and wondering what to do next. Do I ring Elizabeth now and tell her, or wait until after she finishes work? I thought, "This isn't that bad, I'll be OK, and it is treatable". Then I thought, "How dare I be so selfish and not tell her right now. This is something that affects both of us in so many ways". But how the hell do you tell someone you love that you have just been given what immediately comes to mind as being a *death sentence*?

I walked around the house some more, half crying, half resolute. "What do I do next? How can I be rational about a cancer diagnosis?" I went outside to the backyard again, mustered up every ounce of courage, decided to put on my big girl undies (so to speak, not literally) and called Elizabeth at work.

The phone rang and rang, and finally clicked over to leaving a message. She was not answering. "What now? Leave a message? Can't do that. Hang up? Can't do that. Ask her to call me back? Yes". I tried to sound normal, but I don't think I succeeded. In between the phone call, awaiting a response and thinking what to do next, I aimlessly wandered around the house attempting to process the information. Then my phone rang and it was Elizabeth.

To this day, I still don't know exactly what I said. It was something to do with getting pathology results, being diagnosed with endometrial cancer and needing to have a CT scan. I knew I had to emphasise to Elizabeth as quickly as possible that *it was treatable*. Carmel had said it was treatable – so that had to be good, right?

Elizabeth left work immediately to come home. One of her work colleagues generously offered to drive her. It would be about a 30 minute wait. What was I to do? How could I exist in that waiting time? I knew I had to tell someone else and that person had to be someone who could take the emotion out of it for me at this stage and just hear me out.

So I rang a work colleague and said I needed to talk. Eileen was my friend, a nurse, and I knew she would understand because she was aware of what I had been going through for the past few months. As I was blubbering through my tears, I told her about the phone call from my surgeon and that I had been "diagnosed with endometrial cancer". It was so hard to say, but even though it was tough to utter those words, I found this shifted the impact off me in some way. Someone else was now in the loop.

The greatest thing for me was that within a few seconds of telling her the unbelievable and ridiculous news, I was laughing and we were joking together. Yes, this probably was nervous tension and distraction, but it felt good. I told Eileen I was waiting for Elizabeth, so she stayed purposefully on the phone with me until then.

As Elizabeth came walking up the driveway, there I was laughing and being *normal*. This felt absolutely wonderful as a brief moment of being in control, because I knew that over the next few weeks and months there would be many times of feeling out of control. Life was about to be full of unknowns and would be much tougher than usual.

I opened the door and as we embraced, tears gushed down our faces and words were not easy to find. I knew in that moment the only thing making this situation more bearable was that I had the support of my beautiful wife.

Chapter 2

Yellow Star-flyer

This book has evolved from all the pain, trauma, heartache, learning and insight which began from this life-changing, uncontrollable moment. It is also intertwined with my experiences of life to date. These include my upbringing, my successes, my failures, and who I am as a person.

As a past elite athlete for New Zealand, an educator and performance coach in authentic leadership, I now had to draw on every ounce of skill and expertise I possessed to practise what I teach - to thrive and flourish through adversity.

My response to this moment was paramount. I could either buckle and be destroyed by the enormity of it, or I could face it head on and walk into it. The exciting part (even though it may seem strange) of walking through adversity is that this authentic approach works like an absolute genius!

It's about being real, genuine and honest about feeling the emotions of the situation, knowing one's strengths to bring forward, and then devising a plan to move through it. This approach builds on past experiences, knowledge and skills of how to respond to challenges. I have had other moments in my life that were devastating, caused me to feel shock and horror, yet none of them felt like this.

I was privileged to have had a very happy and positive childhood. Both of my parents were extremely supportive of me and would always encourage me to *give things a go*.

Mum would often say, "Just give it a go and then you can properly say whether you like it or not". Dad in his 6-foot 3-inch stature (190 cm) with a gruff looking face, would just smile and say "Well go on then". I knew they would be there for me no matter what, encouraging, supporting and pushing me to achieve more.

Giving things a go from a young age had me eating all types of foods, participating in different activities, learning about my Scottish heritage, and interacting with people from varied backgrounds. This allowed me to gain a sense that there are many views and approaches to life. Giving things a go quickly taught me that a successful result the first time was not guaranteed, but with persistence, the right mindset, and supportive people around me, I could do anything.

I didn't always follow the rules, and at times when it was needed, I would get an *invisible kick in the pants* to get more out of me. Now Dad had a size 13 foot, so the kick (figuratively speaking) was rather hefty and it certainly did the job!

Mum and Dad have since passed away leaving an amazing legacy of sheer grit and determination, fun, good times, and kind-hearted generosity that spreads far and wide to everyone they encountered.

Resilience was drummed into me from an early age. I literally learned that if I fell off my bike (a yellow star-flyer), I got straight back up and carried on pedalling. I would often be riding fast around Foxton Beach Caravan Camp (where we stayed most weekends), doing jumps over the judder bars on my bike, and more often than not, I would come a cropper on the driveway skinning my knees and elbows.

Guaranteed, there would be Mum or Dad's voice from behind a hedge, out of the awning door or standing right in front of me with a big grin saying, "Come on Bell (the nickname my mum gave me), back up on your bike and carry on". This instilled in me that a little knock, a few stones in the knees or elbows was no reason to stop or give up, no matter how much it hurt. Their example and encouragement allowed me to feel safe and supported - to *give things a go*.

Consequently, I gave many sports a go. I played softball, cricket, and soccer, doing pretty well at all of them. Some might say I was a natural sportsperson.

At 16 my family doctor told me I would have to seriously consider giving up soccer. My right knee was injured and would get worse over time, impacting my performance. After two lots of knee surgery I made my way back to sports, but begrudgingly gave up soccer. At the same time the school hockey team needed a goalkeeper. I thought, "Aaahh you just stand there and kick the ball away from the goal, I can do that". Wow, I certainly got that wrong!

I started playing hockey in my last year of secondary school and thought, "Hey I'm good at this, I could make the representative team". It took hard work, don't get me wrong, countless hours of drills, practice, pain (like the time I learned the hard way that I needed to purchase a female groin protector!), bruises the size of a small dinner plate, injuries, and this was just the beginning.

Deep down I believed that I could make the regional representative team, and did. In my first year of playing hockey I made the Manawatu Women's B Team. This gave me a taste of how exciting it was to train hard, push myself, have huge support from my parents and team mates, and do well at something no matter how much I had to sacrifice. I liked it and carried on. Within one year I was selected to represent New Zealand in indoor hockey, a sporting career that lasted 13 years and took me to Australia, Canada and South Africa to play in many tournaments.

Mum's determination certainly rubbed off on me. She was a wee Scottish 5 foot 2½ inch (157 cm) woman, who ran around on 4-inch stilettos, yelling encouragement at the top of her voice to support me and my team. My stoic Dad would always be there behind my goal, mostly quiet until crucial, poignant moments when he would utter a thoughtful word of wisdom to one of us.

I learned through playing sport that *yes* there will be disappointments, losses and devastating moments, but no matter what we think we should or shouldn't be entitled to, the only thing we can control is the way we react to the situation we are in.

I remember early on in my hockey career when I wasn't selected as the number 1 goalie for a team (I was number 2), one of my coaches saying to me, "Ah well, that's the way it is". I NEVER accepted this to be true. I put in many extra hours of training and halfway through that season I was number 1 goalie in that team, and maintained it from then on.

If you saw me on the hockey turf I was formidable. I had learned to be totally focused, show no mercy, and back my team to the fullest. This was a total contrast to me as an extremely shy child, where I would not say boo to anyone or anything. I never spoke up in class, I was too embarrassed to read out loud, and I was never accepted in any group.

I was a loner and in some strange way, felt comfortable with this, knowing that Mum and Dad had my back, and that they supported me to give anything a go.

I developed a strong sense of self-belief and perseverance which became part of my innate strength, my attitude, and actions in life. When things didn't go my way or I did not get the outcome I expected, it was no reason to stop or give up. I became more determined to keep going.

There was always so much more to experience and always a way to get through the tough times. During this sporting period of my life I learned that *my tank* was so much deeper, bigger and more resilient than I ever thought possible. This realisation gave me the foundation to launch into life with unprecedented fervour.

This is what shaped me to cope with my uncontrollable moment that I remember like it was yesterday. That moment on the phone that resulted in shock, terror, surprise, devastation and disbelief. It was like no other I had ever experienced. I had dreams and amazing things I wanted to do and share with people, and then this happened.

From a part, deep down inside of me (my mother's wisdom), came the words she would often say in her warm, Scottish reassuring voice, "Oh well, the sun will still shine tomorrow".

This was the adage that turned me around from focusing on the negatives, looking at the losses, thinking only of the unknown ahead of me, to thinking and asking myself, "What can I do to maintain *ME* on this roller coaster that was about to take off? How can I still enjoy moments and be *present* without my head running off into the dark scary places of the shame and fear around a cancer diagnosis?"

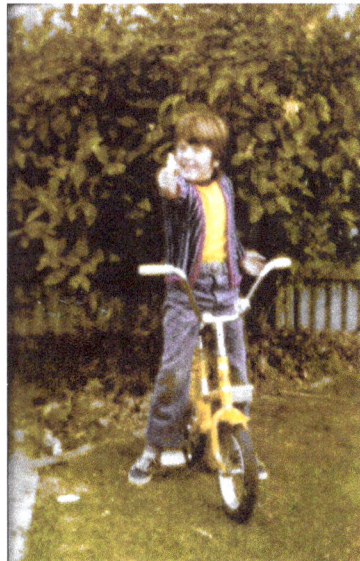

Riding my favourite
Yellow star-flyer bike

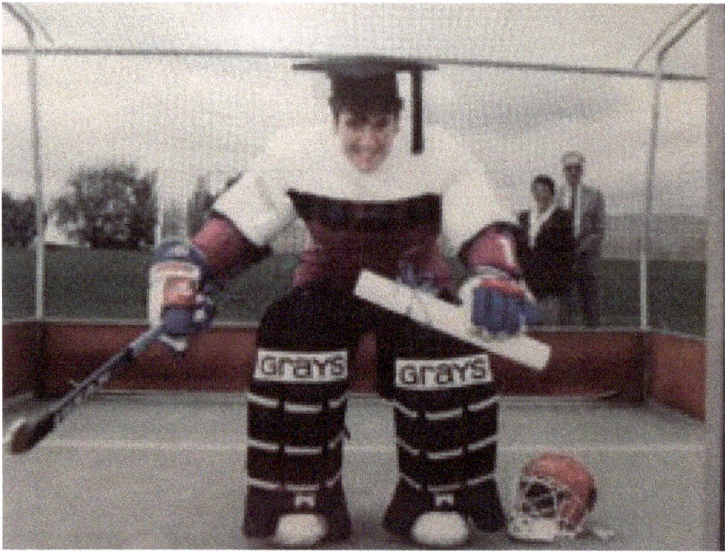

University Graduation photo at Manawatu
Hockey Turf with Mum and Dad

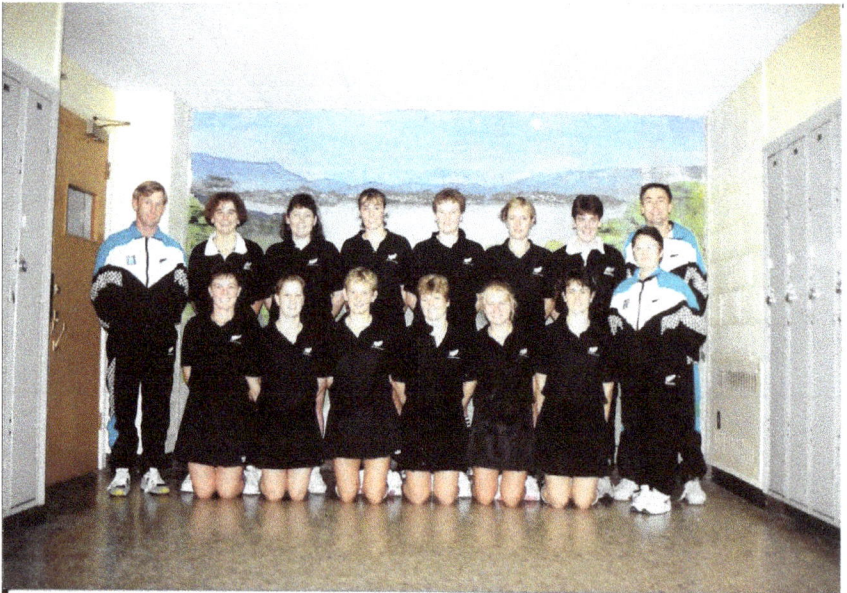

New Zealand Indoor Hockey Team Tour to Canada 1995

CHRISTINE BURNS

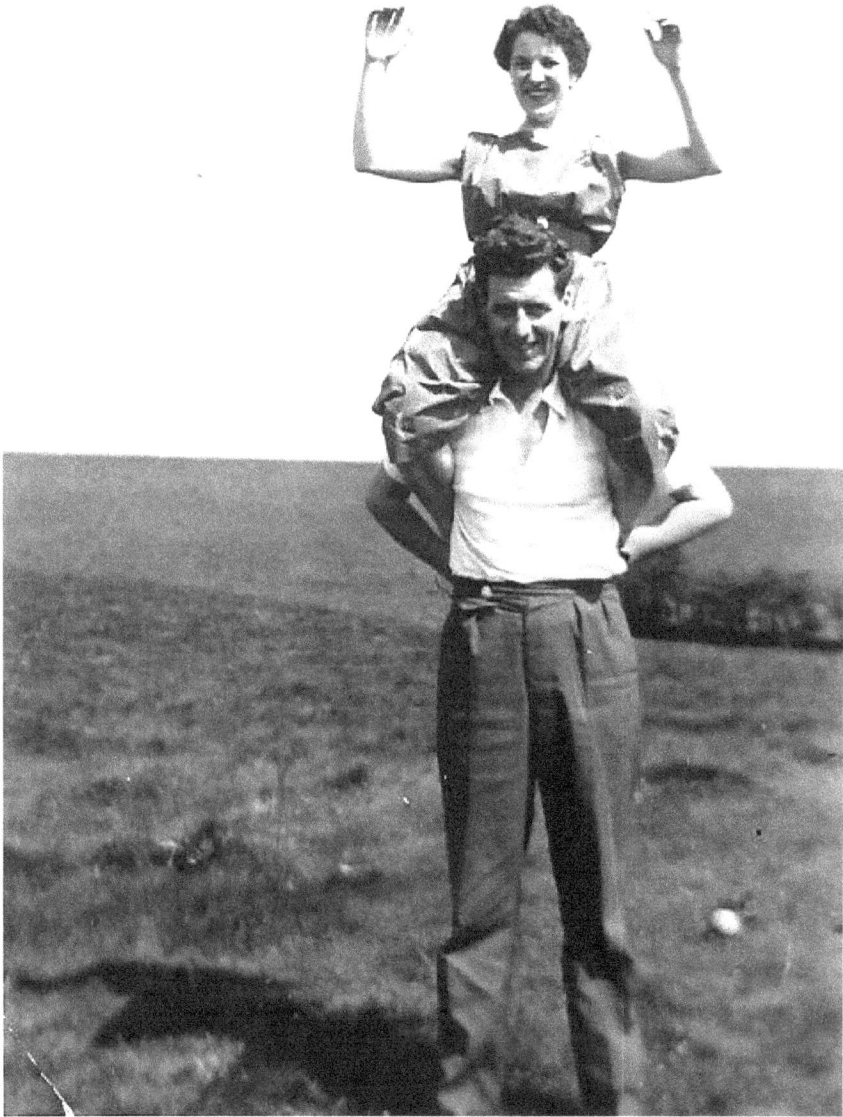

Mum and Dad always having fun

Chapter 3

Roller Coasters

M y emotions were up and down. One minute I was thinking of the worst-case scenario, "I'm too young to die, I haven't finished what I came here to do, I want to do so much more and leave a legacy in this world, how dare anyone or anything think it can come into my body and take over".

The next minute I was thinking rationally and feeling slightly calmer, forcing a smile on my dial, and breathing normally. I found it very important in these moments to be real and honest with myself about the situation as it really was. The term *as-is* has been something I have embraced and used throughout my life. It's about recognising the situation in all its rawness without filters, and understanding my reaction in the moment.

This was reflected in my *nano tanty* as I allowed myself to experience the realness of the situation - the raw emotions of shock, fear and anger. I began thinking "I've got this, they (the medical team) can do their thing medically and I'll do my thing mentally, physically and emotionally".

　　　　　　　　　CHRISTINE BURNS

Just as I was starting to feel on top of these emotions another negative, scary, worrying thought would run through my head and I'd feel the surge of adrenaline again.

"How was I supposed to cope with this event in a country that is not my *home*? What happens next?" I was now living in Australia. In between the questions, I kept repeating the words I heard so clearly, "It is treatable". These three small words gave me the little ray of sunshine I so desperately needed.

The choices and actions I made after that initial phone call were an important step in the game plan. Following my automatic response of having a *nano tanty* and explosion of emotions, my next choice was to hook into my resilient, persevering self and consider the longer-term outcomes with grit and determination.

The emotions of fear, shock, horror and disbelief were coursing through my veins during this acute response phase and I was left with the decision of whether to ruminate on these and allow them to take over, or take control over what I could. I knew I had to physically move because that always assists me to change my headspace in order to think positively and rationally, so that's why I paced around in and out of the house. I decided to get support by contacting people I trusted to express my real thoughts and feelings. I knew that the choices I made in that moment, even though they were uncomfortable, would influence the outcome of future events.

The roller coaster of experiencing emotional ups and downs during challenging events is identified by Roy Baumeister (a Social Psychologist who specialises in willpower, self-control, and self-esteem), as a normal human behaviour (Baumeister & Tierney, 2011).

The ups and downs occur when our negative or *bad* thoughts and feelings override the positive or *good* ones. Evolutionary psychology shows us that human beings have a strong tendency to be attuned to the dangerous or negative things in life in order to survive. Historically this is our protector mechanism, which is extremely necessary for life.

Mihaly Csikszentmihalyi (Professor of Psychology who recognised the concept of 'flow' - a highly focused mental state) discusses the idea that unless we are trained to be preoccupied with positive thoughts, then worrying is our brain's natural default position (2011). We are more likely to notice the danger in situations in order to protect ourselves from potential harm. Even though worrying is the natural tendency for most, there is hope. We can still change this negative response by engaging our willpower, self-control, and self-awareness, choosing a different response to ups and downs.

As human beings we often take the option of catastrophising thoughts and assumptions in a crisis. In times of shock, fear, or extreme worry, we let our thinking explode into a sea of negatives, and things become huge and overwhelming.

Catastrophising happens when we permit ourselves to sink further into negative uncontrollable thoughts, justify poor decision-making habits, or seek to gain attention from others around us.

We often become complacent with the ease of catastrophising and it can become a familiar repeated behavioural pattern. There are ways to shift out of this catastrophising behaviour and make better choices. This needs a certain level of self-awareness in order to adapt our response and break the pattern. Just as we permit ourselves to slide down into the uncontrollable thoughts and engage in poor decision-making, we can become aware of our thoughts, gain clarity over our decisions, and ignite our self-control and willpower.

The first step is to acknowledge the situation *as-is* by verbalising the feelings it is conjuring up. We need to identify the realness of events without hiding or denying the good and the bad. The thoughts we have become, the words we use. When the words we use are negative, irrational

CHRISTINE BURNS

or unfavourable, our emotions will follow, and the actions we choose match this downward spiral.

One of the keys for dealing with an uncontrollable moment is to be present. To be totally in the now. Worrying about what happened in the past, or what might occur in the future is futile. We are not currently in the past, and we are not able to control the future either. We are here, in this moment, this time, this experience. Reflecting on old negative stories and past events in this moment depletes our energy, confuses our head space and affects our ability to take control at that specific point in time.

If we focus on the *what-ifs* or possibilities that may occur in the future, we get distracted and are unable to perform at our best in that moment. When we are immersed in the present moment of time, we are unable to worry about what others may think or how they may react. We are able to focus on what is before us so we can perform at our peak. We need to be present in our own game of life regardless if the situation is familiar or not.

As I woke on Friday 11th November, 2016 I could hear Elizabeth typing furiously on the computer keyboard. She was constructing what I soon realised was our story to share. I didn't want to share anything, as talking about the diagnosis made it more real. I wanted to deal with this on our own, to not show weakness, but realised that we needed help, to build our team. Elizabeth was creating a way for me to be vulnerable, to open up to others, to ask for their help to support me and walk with me through this journey. She created a GoFundMe® campaign. I was unable to work and Elizabeth was part-time and would need to care for me through treatment and recovery.

This campaign took a huge amount of courage and bravery (vulnerability). It epitomised a struggle of realism vs secrecy, health vs ill-health, capability vs incapability. I was worried that my reputation as a strong, competent, healthy person would be compromised. I didn't want people to think I was *sick*, or that I was any less of a person. I didn't want them to put me in the *she has cancer* box and treat me like I was on my death bed. It was making things public putting it out there. It was being vulnerable.

Reading the typed words on the page and creating the beginning of the GoFundMe® post together was difficult for us both. Through the tears we worked through the wording and knew this was a poignant moment. I had been struggling with the idea of telling different people, repeating myself over and over again, and exposing my vulnerable soul. I had been given this diagnosis and was grappling with the idea of who do I tell and how do I tell them?

Dear family and friends (and those we don't yet know),

As many of you know Christine was recently diagnosed with endometrial cancer (at 44) – which was a huge shock as no signs of this were identified previously. She has been unable to work in her role as lecturer at University and has no additional leave to take and is struggling to relieve the pressure of day to day living so that she can focus with lightness on her recovery and upcoming additional surgery and treatment.

She has also recently co-founded a new business that focusses on empowering people to identify their strengths and lead themselves and others with authenticity through finding their passion, ways of creating peak performance and how they can profit in all areas of their life including health, wealth and relationships. This comes from her extensive background in sport and positive psychology, exercise science and her honest realism and desire for people to make changes in their lives to experience higher levels of success.

As a previous elite athlete for New Zealand (indoor and outdoor hockey for 13 years) slowing down physically is not something that comes naturally. She has already shown huge tenacity and resilience over the past few weeks of treatment but needs your help.

We have been so blessed with the warm support we have received and continue to receive from many, and this is what makes the journey bearable and even at times, fun (Christine's two key non-negotiables in life are to have fun, and demonstrate integrity) – however we are asking for some more practical help at this time in order to move the focus from stress to deliberate recovery.

Funds raised by this campaign will go towards immediate medical and living costs towards a full recovery.

By creating the campaign I could get it over with in one click of a button. My intentions for posting were not about stroking my ego, gaining sympathy votes, or getting lots of *likes*. I did it to move one step forward in this journey. It was a way of allowing myself and others to deal with the shocking news. Their response was their choice. I knew I could not control that and was prepared to take the chance.

It was a way of allowing and accepting assistance from people, and showing vulnerability by letting others speak about my life. This was my chance to select my team, and it could not happen until I shared this part of my journey. The uncertainties, assumptions and reservations disappeared with the simple yet courageous action of pressing *post*. This was one of the best actions for me to deal with the diagnosis.

The responses were amazing.

We will never forget the day we went public with this, as we sat together for most of the day reading the numerous written responses of support that flooded in. We alternated between tears of joy, sadness and amazement at the beautiful heartfelt expressions of love and compassion from thousands of friends, loved ones, family, and even strangers across the world.

Putting this out there allowed people to deal with the news in their own way first, then comment, get in touch (or in some cases not), contribute in some way, or watch silently from afar and keep up to date with my journey. These personal contributions have helped ease the trauma of the uncontrollable moment. I am so grateful to all those people who took the time to send well wishes of support to us. The creation of my *team* for this game had begun.

Thank you Elizabeth.

Your limitless possibilities!

1) Call it *as-is*
   - Be real, be true, allow yourself to feel the pain. Be honest with yourself and others.

2) Be aware of your responses
3) Turn your senses on to recognise how you are responding to the situation.
4) Recognise thoughts and choose positive language
   - Think consciously, connect with the self-talk in your head
   - Choose thoughts and words that positively serve you. For me these were: "I CAN do this", "I will be okay", "It's all good", "I've got this"
5) Stay present in the moment
   - Pause, stop, breathe, feel what is happening in the moment (positive AND negative)
   - Use all your senses
6) Be vulnerable
7) Be open and share what you are going through - choose with wisdom who you disclose this to
8) Elicit support
   - You need a team around you that gives you the necessary positive support (this is not sympathy, but strong, realistic encouragement and honest help)
9) Remember what has worked in the past and bring this through (grit and willpower)
   - Look back over events where you have moved through them
   - Identify the things you did, felt, and the thoughts that worked
   - Take ONE thing from this list to implement into your life TODAY, and build it into your daily consistent habits.

Section Two

NOTHING NORMAL

* * *

Affirmation: "I have access to limitless possibilities"

Chapter 4

Hurricane on Steroids

T hree hours after receiving THE phone call, I lay motionless on a CT scanning bed. Breathing in and out as instructed by a mechanical voice. Lying there alone (as no one else was permitted to be in the room) one week after major surgery, restrained by immobilising and positioning blocks, I realised this was one of those times that I needed to allow myself to feel fear. This moment was real. My life had now changed forever. I had just been diagnosed with cancer! This was something to be afraid of.

It was only three hours before that I'd received the phone call that blasted fear into my life like a hurricane on steroids. In the room on my own, I was thinking to myself, "I am so sh*t scared". Scared of what *might* happen, scared of what lay ahead for treatment, scared that they were going to find the cancer had spread to other parts of my body. I was scared that this would be the beginning of the end. The way this scenario was to play out was totally unknown. I had NEVER been this scared in my entire life.

I knew that no matter what they found or what they saw on the CT scan, there was nothing I could do to change the reality of the situation. I couldn't magically make the cancer cells disappear, although I wanted to with every ounce of strength in my body. I struggled with the fact they could see the results on their screens and I couldn't. I had to wait the interminable, undefined amount of time before I was privy to them. I couldn't believe this was happening to ME!

So many thoughts raced through my head at the time. "I am fit and healthy, there's no logical reason why I should have something like this happen to me. I can't believe I've been dealt this crap in life". This alternated with curiosity about how the machine worked, and what the staff were doing in their little room. I was then jolted back into the moment by the electronic voice telling me to breathe again. Breath in and hold; more thoughts; "Why is this happening, I don't deserve this?", followed by more noise, spinning, thoughts, feelings - overwhelm. ARGH!

There was no way I could eliminate this diagnosis from my life. I couldn't ignore it, I couldn't deny it, I couldn't change it. It was real! Would I need further surgery, radiotherapy, or chemotherapy? What would my treatment and prognosis be? These questions were the unknown, which had become the uncontrollable, and I needed some answers.

My next appointment didn't answer all of these questions. Although I did get one answered. I needed radiotherapy and would receive tattoos at a simulation session for accuracy and alignment of the treatment. There was a part of me that was curious and intrigued about this simulation and tattooing session. What happens in a simulation? How did they do the tattoos? How big would they be? Why does everything need to be such a step-by-step process? I soon found out.

The simulation session involved lots of measuring, small adjustments of how I was positioned on the table, with laser lights and tape measures adjusting my placement, tattoos etched in four places, and lying very still the entire time allowing the radiographers to do their thing. I found having the tattoos weird, interesting, and also a tad daunting knowing they were a permanent reminder of what was being done.

During this appointment, which could have been very scary and stressful, I stayed in the moment, chatted with the therapists, asked questions, and learned more about the process with a few laughs along the way. It helped to put us all at ease, and it was actually in the weirdest way a fun experience.

The thing that hit me like a ton of bricks was when I was called through to begin the simulation session, Elizabeth had to stay in the small waiting room. I had now begun this daunting and incongruent routine of walking off with these medical people into the unknown without my support, someone that I knew would have my back and so dearly wanted to be right beside me. Those next few steps were tough to take, as I knew I had just gone to another level in this journey. In my head was, "This sh*t just got real".

The other interventions and prognosis were still an unknown. My team were unsure if I would need chemotherapy until I had more tests, including a Positron Emission Tomography (PET) scan. The PET scan involved being injected with a radioactive tracer. Just the name of it sounded scary. This fluid was so dangerous that the staff needed to be fully protected with an apron, thick gloves, eye protectors, and had to stand away from the injecting apparatus at the end of the bed behind a protective wall. The fluid was encased in a lead radioactive protection container to reduce the risk of contaminating staff or others in the area.

The staff were only allowed to perform three of these administrations a day due to the toxicity of the fluid, but here I was, having this toxic fluid injected into MY veins, and I still had no idea what the outcome would be. I was then instructed to lay motionless for **one whole hour** so the toxic tracer could find its mark.

This procedure was yet another source of fear along this unwanted journey. The only way I knew how to handle this tough situation was to work out how to take control, even for a small part of it. I was given a choice of what movie to watch from the bed, so I chose "Despicable Me" - the children's movie.

I have always loved children's movies and find the humour and silliness of them to be refreshing. I figured if I had to lie still for an hour, I might as well be in the moment and have some fun. Finding a moment of *normality* whilst lying in the lead-lined room waiting for a PET scan, was important for me.

Part of the PET scan preparation was a trip to the bathroom, when I experienced a moment that totally jolted me from my self-absorption. It occurred when I was walking between rooms. The door to the PET scanner opened and I saw a young girl about seven years old, with a bald head, come out through the door. She was smiling and chatting with the staff as she walked towards her dad, who was waiting for her. It was obvious that she was in the chemotherapy phase of treatment for childhood cancer. It seemed like she was just taking the moment in her stride, having a giggle with the staff as she walked out, and they treated her with respect and tender care.

Her dad had a remorseful look on his face, one that displayed a mix of emotions. Smiling to comfort his daughter, yet enmeshed with uncertainty and tinged with the faint ardour of "This is so unfair, this is not right!"

It gave me a huge lump in my throat and I felt what could only be described as one of those hard belly punches. You know, the one that stops you mid-stride, takes your breath away and leaves you gasping for air. A feeling which I later found out would arise many times throughout this journey.

It seemed so unfair for any child to go through this, and it was not right or fair for me either. On the other hand, it was encouraging to see this wee girl, as it tended to put things into perspective for me. I had already lived five times longer on this planet than she had. I had the tools and skills to work with this, and I needed to step up and handle it the best way I knew how. If this little girl could be happy while handling this situation, then I could too.

The wait for the radiotherapy sessions began. The chasm of the 47 days between the initial diagnosis phone call to the first radiotherapy treatment was like a living hell. At times I didn't know which way was up. Would I be alive this time next year, what would I be able to do during the treatment, and what sort of condition would I be in after the treatment?

I was still recovering from major surgery and very limited with what I could do physically each day. The thing I found the toughest was that I had no idea what I was *meant* to be doing or feeling. I was in pain, restricted with physical movements; unable to drive; unable to lift; unable to work; financially pressured and receiving unhelpful responses from my boss; feeling like a burden on my partner; confused emotionally and mentally as there were no definite timeframes, no obvious outcomes and no specific rules to live through this. I was still me. Nothing had changed yet everything had changed. I was dangling in limbo land!

My first radiotherapy session was scary! More unknowns. I had no idea what was planned for me and this freaked me out, never mind the fact that I was going into the Peter MacCallum Cancer Centre section of the hospital. I turned left at the hospital entrance. A turn that no-one ever wanted to take.

My first radiotherapy appointment was at the end of the day at 4pm. It seemed like everything that day moved in slow motion and lasted forever. It was long and drawn out before the time to drive to the hospital finally arrived. This was the beginning of what would become a routine for the next five weeks (25 sessions).

On the way to the hospital I was on autopilot. Going through the paces without knowledge of what was happening. Elizabeth drove and I sat motionless in the passenger seat. My heart rate was high, my palms were sweaty, and I was only breathing because my body made it happen automatically. My head was all over the place. I wasn't quite sure how I actually got to the door of the hospital from the carpark. I do remember walking into the hospital and thinking "Oh my gosh, I have to do the walk of shame and turn left into the Peter Mac wing, the CANCER wing". My thoughts and feelings were racing off into their own crazy, irrational story.

We walked in, turned left, my heart skipped a few beats. My breathing stopped for what seemed like an age as we walked through the double doors towards the reception desk. As a sportsperson this was a whole new *game* for me, and I was out of my depth. I didn't know the formal rules of this game, and I hadn't been able to establish any of my own informal rules or work out the usual behaviours of the team. I was the newbie, the nervous looking one.

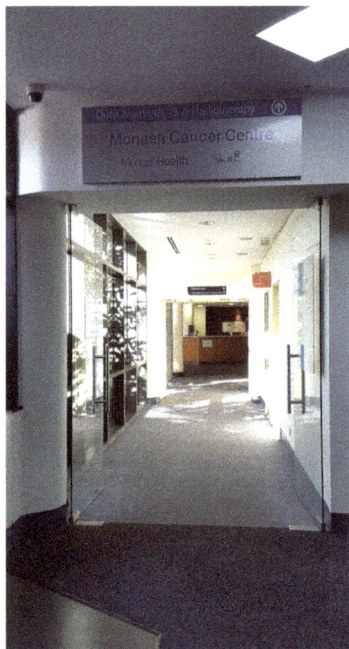

Turning Left towards the Peter Mac Moorabbin Cancer Centre.

As we checked in and scanned my electronic card, my name popped up on the computer screen letting the radiation therapists know I was in the building. The receptionist pointed to a dark enclosed room (the waiting room). She told us to take a seat there and one of the therapists would be with us shortly. The room oozed fear, anxiety, trauma, and cancer.

We both walked to the entrance of this room and then stopped abruptly and turned around. It was like hitting a brick wall. We just stood there wide eyed, motionless. Elizabeth asked if we could sit over in the other waiting area that was bright and open. The answer was a definitive NO! That bright, open waiting room was for a different section of the hospital. The dark enclosed waiting room was the specific area for the cancer patients waiting for radiotherapy, and that was now me.

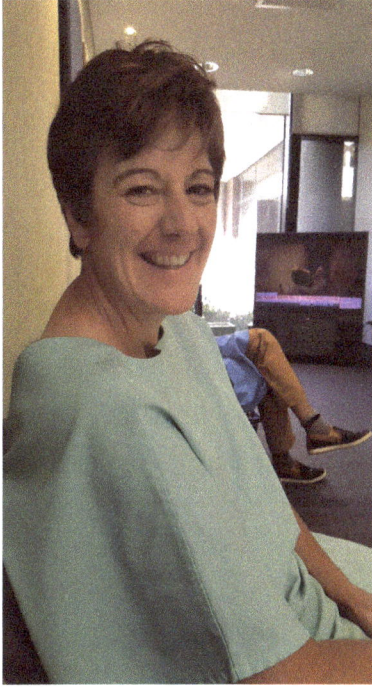

I sat in the waiting room looking and listening to what was going on around me. I had a sense of hypervigilance. Acutely aware of the sounds, smells, and the feeling of the place. My name was called. I shot up out of my seat, full of nervous energy, with a smile on my dial (a nervous one) and greeted the first of many of my new *team mates*.

All gowned up and ready to begin first day of radiation treatment.

As the radiation therapist introduced herself and described where we were walking off to, all I could hear was my own heart pounding in my ears. At this stage, I was given a gown, instructions on the *rules*, and told I would be given 30 (not 25) treatment sessions. What? She just said 30 treatments! Another unknown, and another cause for fear.

Did they know something I didn't? Did I have a worse diagnosis than I initially understood? Why had the *rules* changed on me?

And so the routine began ... from the dark front room around to the back waiting area, collect my gown from my personally named tray (from the many cupboards holding other people's gowns), grab a basket from the pile, go to the cubicle, get changed into my gown, put my street clothes into the basket, and take a seat. Another waiting game until it was time for me to proceed down yet another corridor and take my place on the radiotherapy bed.

Walking into that room for the first time and being confronted with a machine that resembled a massive *transformer*, was a sight that is etched into my brain. I must admit, for a few seconds curiosity and intrigue kicked in and I became fascinated at how the machine did its job. Then I had a moment of complete consciousness, feeling totally vulnerable as I stood there at the entrance of the room in my light green gown, totally on my own. It was like a shot from a movie where everything is huge and I was just a tiny image surrounded by light, walking into the dark unknown area with the transformer.

In writing this I was reminded that I wasn't alone. Elizabeth informs me that she was there and so were the two radiation therapists. It felt like I was alone, scared, and walking into the world of further unknown. It's strange how we remember things differently from what they actually were. I was looking down the barrel of a massive transformer, thinking I had entered into yet another experience that was absolutely foreign to me and darn right scary. The next step of my new routine continued.

I got onto the table of the transformer and it was time for them to switch on the electronic lasers. These aligned with my tattoo markers and then positioning blocks were set in place. Once I was positioned correctly, the therapists left the room and told me not to move. I was on my own again, motionless, hardly daring to breathe until I received the next instruction. This lasted about 20 minutes each time, while the radiation therapists were next door operating the machine remotely.

They were able to see my every move on video cameras, and hear every breath through several microphones dotted around the room. As I lay on the treatment bed while the machine buzzed, whirred and creaked around me, I could see the transformer lurching above me as if it was alive. This was terrifying yet intriguing. How can something so big, and so plastic-looking be so technologically advanced with the laser focus precision to kill cancer cells?

Playing sport had taught me how to shift my focus from the emotional happenings to the technical and objective side of situations. Even though I had been trained to shift my focus quickly, and maintain high levels of precision in moments of apprehension or fear in sport, I was only able to maintain this focus for a few minutes during that first session.

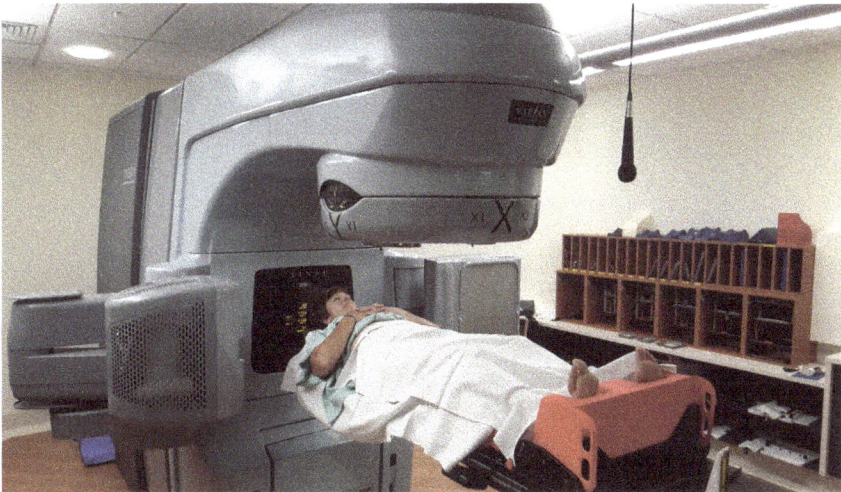

Lying as still as possible controlling the controllables, receiving radiation treatment.

Reflecting on the first scan and the first radiotherapy session while writing this section of the book, brought me to tears. This was still so real, so vivid and so memorable. I realised that I could not run from the situation. The words of the diagnosis continue to confront me each and every day - I had just been diagnosed with cancer. I still have feelings of fear, lack of control, and experience times of being thrust into the unknown.

At every follow-up appointment I thought, "So what happens today?" I have so many skills and abilities in multiple areas to deal with new situations in life, but I have absolutely no control over this health diagnosis. I cannot predict what each day will bring or what the outcome will be. Living with the unknown, living with fear had become a daily game requirement.

Chapter 5

Anatomy of Fear

*So, what is fear? A natural reaction
to the unknown, isn't it?*

Fear is defined in the American Psychological Association dictionary as a "basic, intense emotion aroused by the detection of imminent threat, involving an immediate alarm reaction that mobilises the organism by triggering a set of physiological changes" (2016).

Fear is a feeling induced by a perceived danger or threat that occurs, causing a change in behaviour. It is a perception of a situation or a response to an experience. The way I perceive this situation right now is based on information and social perception that people have reported following a cancer diagnosis. This is usually negative.

An unknown situation + standing in front of a transformer that annihilates cancerous cells = Fear!

Fear is a natural response, a natural psychological warning system that happens inside our brains. It keeps us safe. It stops us from taking risks that are dangerous (walking in front of a car), and it notifies us when there is potential to get hurt (keeping away from the edge of a cliff). In response to this situation, I was experiencing a great deal of fear. "Will I get hurt? Is it dangerous? Am I safe? Will I still be alive in one years' time?"

Fear is a reaction we all experience at times in our lives. It often goes hand-in-hand with anxiety. As soon as we feel fear, the amygdala (a small almond-shaped organ in the centre of the brain) sends out a warning signal to the autonomic nervous system (ANS). The ANS is a control system that acts largely unconsciously and regulates bodily functions such as heart rate, digestion, respiratory rate, pupillary response, urination, and sexual arousal. In times of fear and anxiety (also known as *stress*) the heart rate rises, breathing quickens, and stress hormones such as adrenaline and cortisol are released throughout the bloodstream.

The blood in the torso is redirected from the heart to the extremities (arms and legs). This prepares the body for action, and results in the brain functioning on automatic. The ability to think, reason, and problem solve decreases. Planning the next move, or deciding how to do it, is impaired.

The common understanding in psychology is that the more stressed a person is, the *dumber* they are, i.e. they make silly decisions. The positive by-product of this level of stress is that it assists with a heightened sense of alertness, leading to the intention of maintaining survival.

There are common physical responses to fear and stress as the ANS kicks in and prepares the body for *fight or flight*. One response is sweating. Sweating may be interpreted as *bad* however it helps to cool the body and it regulates body temperature – this is *good*. A great way to look at this is that the body is responding positively to prepare for participation in the *game of life*.

A pounding heart is often felt or heard as a response to fear. This heavy pounding is the body's release of adrenaline, which increases the blood flow around the body to the working muscles. Feeling the heart pounding in the chest or hearing it in the ears is a sign that the body has increased strength and energy for what lies ahead. Increased power to do what is required.

When we realise that our response to stress is protective and positive for saving our lives, then we can change our perception around these responses which will ease the angst. Another reaction is the tight feeling around our chest and shoulders, which is the body preparing for survival. This tightening also increases the respiration rate. The increased rate is providing more oxygen to fuel the muscles and brain with oxygenated blood to create clarity of thought and speedy reactions.

An additional response in the face of fear is a dry mouth or throat. The body is working automatically and is in survival mode, therefore will divert any non-essential fluids towards the action-taking zones. The need for talking or having moist lips has been relegated to the bottom of the list, as the need for survival takes precedence. These reactions to stress are often seen as a negative consequence. However, these reactions are hugely positive as they are protecting you, helping your body to be efficient in the situation and therefore must be embraced and not feared.

Franklin Roosevelt knew the destructive nature of fear. As the 32nd President of the United States (1933-1945), he chose his words very carefully when he told the nation that was in the grips of the Great Depression and looming World War: "We have nothing to fear but *fear* itself."

Fear makes things worse. It serves no purpose. If we can control our fears, we can regain control of that moment by recognising what is happening and identifying what is going on. Label the emotion(s) and work out what will support you. Is the fear creating adrenaline in your body to propel you forward in a positive way, or is it tripping you up? If it's the latter, then you need to let go of the emotion and walk through it. This is the first step towards creating a fuller, more satisfying life. Fear is a perception. Shifting, changing or re-interpreting this perception gives rise to a more effective outcome.

Fear is one of the many emotions that may appear during the tough times, but it may also be accompanied by anger or guilt. These emotions may feel uncomfortable and even painful. But remember, emotions are just feedback. They are internal data that can be incredibly useful to us. Emotions are on a continuum and they are dynamic. When we recognise our emotions and don't get scared by the *negative* ones, we can use them for good.

Fear does not have to be a bad thing. Being scared does not have to be a bad thing. Emotions can be neutral. We assign meaning to these emotions that often aren't necessary. We tend to want to run away from the tough ones. However, we can come through the situation, learn from it and use the emotions as data to drive us forward.

Dr Robert Biswas-Diener is widely known as the *Indiana Jones of psychology* for his research on happiness and emotions. His work takes him to adventurous places such as Greenland, Kenya and India, interviewing disparate communities including Amish farmers, sex workers in Kolkata, peace protesters in Palestine, and the Maasai Tribe.

He has identified that our entire range of emotions is essential when responding to threats and getting through all life events, no matter how big or traumatic the event may seem. We cannot disregard or shy away from emotions, but embrace them all in order to find a way through any event that comes our way.

In their book titled 'The Upside of Your Dark Side', Kashdan and Biswas-Diener (Professor of Psychology at George Mason University and a world recognised authority on wellbeing; and positive psychologist, author and instructor at Portland State University) explored the requirement to recognising and embracing the whole of self - the complete range of emotions (2014). The dark and the good sides drive us to achieve success and fulfillment in all areas of our lives. If a person avoids emotions like negativity, fear, and anxiety they will miss out on the benefits of being a *whole* person. They will not be able to recognise the good stuff.

If we numb what we interpret as bad or difficult, then we also numb the ability to feel excitement, joy and elation. That's the way it works. Many of us want to push the negative stuff aside and pretend that it doesn't exist. But we cannot have one without the other. A person who experiences both positive and negative emotions harnesses the power of being themselves. They are more resilient, healthier, happier and able to reach their full potential without any blocks. This is termed *psychological flexibility*.

When a person is psychologically (emotionally) flexible and able to feel and embrace the complete range of emotions, they are psychologically healthy. They are able to cope with the tough times. They recognise how to express emotions, have less stress, sleep better and are more engaged in the world around them, even during times of great adversity. This emotional flexibility is the key.

Most people during times of adversity search for a way to feel a small window of brightness or joy in times of hardship. Some call this happiness. I know we did. Being aware that happiness is more than the pursuit of all things good (an impossibility), or a fleeting moment of pleasure, psychologists Ed Diener of the University of Illinois at Urbana-Champaign and Shigehiro Oishi of the University of Virginia, set about to explore what made people happy. They conducted research with more than 140,000 participants from 132 countries (Oishi & Diener, 2013). They asked people to rate happiness in comparison to other highly desirable personal outcomes.

For example, having meaning in life, becoming rich, and getting into heaven. They found that the most psychologically healthy people didn't deny their own feelings or ignore them. Psychologically healthy people were able to express anger, were more comfortable with negative states of emotion, and were effective in dealing with life's ups and downs. These people viewed emotions not as negative or positive, but as blended states. They recognised that a person can be afraid and curious at the same time, or anxious and excited simultaneously.

Psychologically healthy individuals have the ability to tolerate discomfort, and depending on their circumstances and environment, are able to shift to a different place in their head (change their mindset), which allows them optimal results in every situation. Anger fuels creativity, guilt sparks improvement, self-doubt enhances performance, and selfishness increases courage. When we embrace the entirety of our emotional state with flexibility then we become astute and aware individuals who are resilient and empowered, able to forge ahead and flourish with joy and contentment.

Happy, flourishing people don't hide from negative emotions. They acknowledge that life is full of disappointments and fear, then either find a way through them or face them head on. An individual who is flourishing in life may use feelings of anger or guilt as a motivator to effectively change their behaviour. This agile mental shifting between pleasure and pain is the ability to modify behaviour to match a situation's demands.

At some point in our lives we all experience trauma. It may affect health, family, finances, or our core instinct to survive. It is quite normal to have a strong emotional or physical reaction following a distressing event. On many occasions these reactions will subside as part of the mental, physical and emotional recovery. Our responses to these events are influenced by our ability to flourish in life and our level of emotional flexibility.

Unfortunately, it often takes something significantly traumatic for us to wake up and realise what really matters in life. It does not need to take the loss of a loved one, a personal health scare, a natural disaster, or financial trauma, to shock us into sitting up and taking notice of the meaning and reason we are here in this world. However, we often ignore the early warning signals that gently nudge us until it becomes undeniable.

When we finally pay attention to the confronting situation, we may recognise our impermanence on this planet and are left with a choice. The choice to either make sense of the situation and find meaning within it, or become a victim to the event and slide down the pathway to personal destruction. Even in the darkest moments we can choose how we show up every day.

The first thing I did each morning (and still do) is smile when I wake up. We can prepare ourselves with a positive intention each day. For me this was having three positive moments within the treatment or outside of it.

We can choose to care for ourselves with the resources, skills and abilities that we have available. I chose a clean, healthy diet without preservatives or sugar. We can choose how we present ourselves. I carefully selected clothing to attend my appointments each day. We can respect others and build connections. I connected meaningfully with people in the waiting room and with the staff. We can choose engagement with others. I chose sharing with vulnerability through fulfilling conversations. We can choose to develop meaning and growth. I chose to learn something new every day and contribute to those closest to me.

Throughout the two months of receiving radiation therapy, there were brief moments when I was able to shift enough fear aside so I could experience being *present*. The doubt, the fear, and the uncertainty would often rise insidiously in the back of my mind. I was recovering from multitudes of medications, transfusions, all types of scans, and two major surgical procedures. My energy, abilities and resolve were well below

100%. It was more like 30%. My usual high degree of emotional and mental strength had been emaciated. My physical capacity was almost non-existent. I needed to find a way to build this potency back up, to create a way forward for the very next day, and also the rest of my life.

There are some rituals and strategies that got me through this time. They kept me safe, gave me a sense of control, and provided a purpose for the day. One of the rituals I worked out early in the treatments was to have my fingers interlaced across my chest. This was practical as it kept my arms away from the machine while it travelled around me. This pose also created a focus for my energy (the top of my body) as the other parts of my body were either immobilised or being treated.

When moving onto the table, I was thinking through my plan and setting myself up to carry out my game. This became part of my *pre-game ritual*, and my mental focus during the treatment each day. I was setting myself up for success mentally and emotionally as I had done many times before when playing hockey. I used this time to silently say to myself, "I am so grateful and thankful now that every cell in my body is healthy and vibrant". I recited this from the moment the radiotherapists left the room until the transformer did its last zap. Every single session, every single minute, every single day. Consistently!

This mantra came from a heartfelt place and was recited with a huge smile. I felt the joy of it. It gave me a sense of purpose, kept me in the present moment and allowed me to focus on healing. I treated this as a sacred time to meditate, to control my breathing, to slow down, to be intrigued by the noises and movement of the giant transformer as it made its way around my body, shuffling, realigning its leaves and healing me.

As I reflect on this now, I see this entire experience as a precious gift through which I have been allowed to learn who I am and what I possess. I don't see this today as a negative or sad thing, although still feel emotional when thinking of this time. In a way I feel grateful that I had this opportunity. It was extremely hard and the toughest challenge I have ever had to face in my life, but the experience has given me many learnings.

There is always more in my tank, there are always people out there who can help, there is always someone else who needs to have a kind word, a laugh or a connection from me. This is not from a space of ego, but I am truly thankful and grateful that I could come through this traumatic event to experience these teachings. I had choices to make every day. The choices I made in thought and action allowed me to move another step towards my purpose.

Although I never asked to be in this situation, being confronted by some of my darkest fears, learning to accept them, deal with them, and make friends with my fears, has enabled me to learn, grow, and bounce forward into my *new normal*.

*"Sometimes amongst the darkest skies, the
brightest stars reveal themselves and shine"*
– Christine Burns –

Chapter 6

New Normal

The elephant in the room that
no-one wanted to talk about.

I had just been given a cancer diagnosis – this was huge and I didn't want to admit it to anyone. In my head was a quick fix to this diagnosis. I would be "outta there" and back to full health before anybody knew it. I didn't need to tell anyone what was going on. Did I?

Of course, it was irrational and a big cover up. I had started to believe my own ludicrous story - that this was something small and I could cope with it on my own. I had developed so many strategies to get on top of things, no matter what the play. But this was an exception to the rule. This denial stemmed from being afraid. When I stopped running from the fear and allowed my heart to go to that scary place, where the unprotected feelings and vulnerability lived, I realised I had no idea what was going on or what would eventually happen to me.

The constant phone calls and appointments with specialists and health services tore down the taboo around discussing cancer. I wanted to pretend it wasn't happening to me, that everything would be fine, but really, I had no idea. It took some time to become aware that the taboo subject I was becoming accustomed to talking about, wasn't happening for other people. Saying the words *cancer diagnosis* was now becoming a familiar part of my vocabulary but I had not yet linked myself with the words or accepted that as part of me.

My struggle with acknowledging the elephant in the room had increased. The daily visits to the Cancer Centre were drilling the word *cancer* into my life. The routines and habits associated with this adversity were becoming a hauntingly familiar part of daily life. When people asked me how I was, I wanted to scream at them, "HOW DO YOU THINK I AM, I HAVE JUST BEEN DIAGNOSED WITH CANCER". The problem was that I didn't know how to respond. Was I meant to let it all out and bombard them with the true realities of how I was feeling, or did I respond politely to make them feel safe and reassure them about the situation?

Gradually I began talking about it. Elizabeth and I needed to have some support as this was beginning to take its toll and we couldn't do it on our own. I couldn't understand why some friends and colleagues ceased contact. They faded away from being an integral part of my life, to not being there at all. Had I missed the memo that cancer had become a communicable disease? Was I contagious? Or were my expectations of acceptance too high? Is there a rule that one does not share their story too widely or speak about these things?

I was beginning to feel isolated. Friends and colleagues no longer asked me how I was; no short messages of acknowledgement or support were received; very few texts or communications from family arrived. I felt as if I had become non-existent and relegated to the too-hard basket.

My workplace was not understanding and treated me as if I had a common cold. Some friends talked about everything else and avoided the subject. Others put on a brave face and pulled out the "Oh well, keep fighting, you're a battler". It was like people were running out of my life when I needed them most. I had just been married six months prior and we were now a bigger family. Very few of them were in touch to see how they could help or contribute.

This even happened for my wife. What broke my heart the most was that many didn't even ask her (their own sibling) how she was doing in this whole topsy-turvy moment that had abruptly taken over our lives with a vengeance. We were living in a new country that had only been our home for five years and we had very few extended networks in place.

These experiences added to the size of the elephant. The strange thing in life is, if you have a broken arm in a cast everyone wants to know what happened. It's a real talking point. They want the whole story with the sequence of events. Having endometrial cancer however, people don't want to know the story, they don't want to ask what happened, they don't want to go there.

One of the strategies I incorporated into my recovery after the initial GoFundMe® post to describe and make sense of the elephant, was to share my diagnosis on Facebook with friends. The post was first and foremost to admit to myself the realness of the situation. This was a huge step. Then to acknowledge that my future was unknown and share this with people who I considered part of my life.

I knew there were many people who found discussing cancer absolutely frightening. I also wanted to be a voice for those people and stand up in solidarity for the *team* I had just become a member of. In my eyes, clicking *post* could not make things worse. I had just been given a diagnosis that was bigger than me, bigger than any social network, and I knew that people would respond in their own way.

I remember telling an acquaintance that I had posted on Facebook about my diagnosis and maintained regular posts through sharing the

GoFundMe® updates each month or so. He laughed at me and proceeded to mock the use of a social media site to open up and share my story. To him sharing personal information was unthinkable in such a public arena. He stated, "Surely there are better ways to get attention". I wanted to punch him in the face for that comment. I was angry. Then self-doubt crept in. Maybe he was right. Will other people think the same? Have I made a stupid mistake?

After much agonising I determined that for me, it was time to open up and let others into my life. The tough guarded exterior I had always publicised had to be abandoned. SCARE FACTOR 10/10! I wanted, in fact I needed, people in my life right now.

The doubt, anger and the scepticism I was experiencing, were gradually washed away by the multitudes of positive and heartfelt messages of support. Connections with people I had not spoken to for years were resurrected, and current friends shared their adverse experiences with me in an in-depth, courageous and respectful way.

This team gave me an additional avenue for me to download, rather than continually burdening and dumping the rawness and uncertainty of the diagnosis on Elizabeth. Our support team had just increased. Heartfelt well wishes from people helped both of us to keep this elephant tamed and at bay.

In many groups and communities it is more acceptable to hide or mask negative feelings, and only share tolerated affirming experiences. It is often easier to minimise the extent of the situation or hide behind the mask of invincibility or stoicism whilst not admitting personal struggles.

The term masking was first used by Paul Ekman, an American psychologist, who consulted with Pixar for the film *Inside Out*. Masking is when an individual conceals one emotion by portraying another emotion. It is mostly used to hide negative emotions (usually sadness, frustration, and anger) with positive emotions (joy, gratitude, or serenity).

Often when we see someone hurting we offer optimism and reassurance to minimise the pain instead of facing the negativity and uncertainty in the moment.

Sheryl Sandberg, Chief Operating Officer of Facebook, highlighted this point as she was dealing with the trauma of her husband's death stating, "Yep, I see a grey animal in the room, but that's no elephant – looks more like a mouse" (Sandberg & Grant, 2017, p.38). She discussed how in an effort to deal with something so immense, she pretended it was smaller than it really was. In that moment it was simpler to downplay the trauma by minimising the size of the elephant, and to mask the impact instead of acknowledging the reality of the situation. We too have the power to interpret the size of the elephant or the mouse in the room at any time.

Struggling to keep a positive mindset

Each day we would arrive at the hospital, enter the front door and take the dreaded left turn to the Peter Mac Cancer Centre. I checked-in electronically and we took our place in the cancer patient area. I often noticed people from the bright open waiting room on the other side looking at us with a troubled look on their faces. What I read in the speech bubbles above their heads was, "Oh my gosh she looks so fit and healthy; why on Earth is she in there", "Thank God it's not me" and "I wonder how much longer she has".

The energy in our waiting room felt sombre, full of fear, and was usually very quiet. It was like walking into a chamber of fragility. It would be so easy to go in feeling anxious, worried and expecting the worst each day. I was so scared to begin with sitting in this waiting room, even with

Elizabeth next to me. We were surrounded by people who looked sad, anxious, angry, desperate or just withdrawn from life. Would being in the waiting room with these people make me sicker? Would I fall victim to the misrepresented perception that having cancer is a death sentence?

Elizabeth and I seized every opportunity we could to lighten up the place, to alleviate this environment of the dis-ease. We would impart our own tipping point - three positive things for one negative - into the room. Could we get three smiles for each frown? Were we able to summon three positive comments from a fellow team mate we sat alongside? I resolved that I would not be influenced by this dark, negative energy in a way that would cause me to be drawn into this dis-ease. I was determined not to let this happen on every level.

The challenge, I now realise, is the human brain is wired towards negativity. It's an evolutionary construct for survival. When the human body experiences adversity, anxiety rises and it is consumed mentally, physically and emotionally by the negativity of the situation. This leaves little to no room for thinking about possible solutions or options.

The famous quote by Henry Ford, "*Whether you think you can or think you can't you're right*", challenged and sustained me throughout my journey. If I were to be angry, closed-minded,

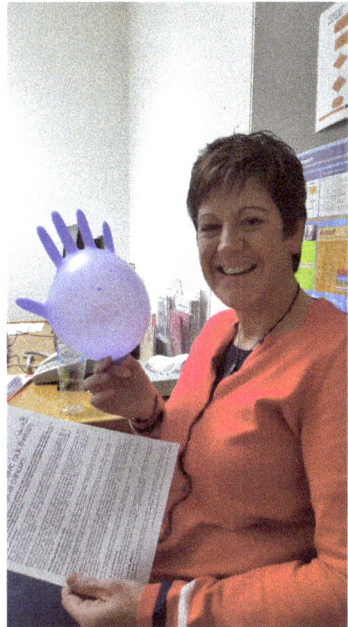

There's always time for fun. Even on the day of getting test results!

intentionally shut people out and sink into a victim mentality, then I would be *right*. I would be and remain negative. This would be detrimental to my wellbeing. The way that I chose my thoughts and actions in this situation was affecting my ability to flourish each day. If I were to be positive, authentic, vulnerable, and open about my situation then I would be *right*.

Eating became a whole new game — what can I eat?

The daily radiotherapy treatment was damaging my gut and diminishing the ability to digest food. As the treatments accumulated it became easier not to eat. There were so many foods my body couldn't tolerate and the discomfort was intensifying. Whenever I was going out and about I was obsessed with knowing where the bathrooms were, just in case my stomach decided it didn't like the food I had eaten.

The radiation therapy, which kills both mutated and healthy cells, was enforcing its side effects – diarrhoea, nausea, vomiting, nutrient malabsorption and dehydration. Cancer cells grow and divide much faster than healthy cells, so the treatment area needed to be larger than where the cancer was discovered. I was diagnosed with endometrial cancer, therefore the area for treatment and damage was the lower abdomen, pelvic area, gastrointestinal tract, bladder and bowel.

My thinking around food choices changed dramatically. Initially I just chose not to eat as it reduced the discomfort and the side effects which were too hard to manage. It was easier not to upset my body. I quickly realised that not eating was totally counterintuitive to a flourishing recovery.

To rebuild the tissue damage from surgery and radiotherapy, I needed to eat healthy foods. To get my energy levels and strength back up, I needed to eat healthy foods. To help me get back on my feet from a year of rapidly declining health, I needed to eat healthy foods. Even when I worked out which foods worked today, tomorrow my body often rejected them. It was tough, confusing and beyond my control. This was compounded by other people's reactions, where some were understanding and others were very critical. Regardless of their response, I needed to get to the point where I understood that these side effects and the discomfort related to food did not define me, and it wouldn't be like this forever.

Dragging myself off the couch

During this time of treatment and recovery, I continued to have a declining amount of energy. Instigating my pre-game routines and my three-to-one strategy, the first two weeks of treatment seemed like I was on a high and able to stay above the side effects of radiotherapy. But as time progressed, the fatigue insidiously crept into every part of my body and life, as more and more of the healthy cells were killed off.

Eventually at the end of treatment my physiological body was in a state of depletion and weakness. I lacked energy on every level, mentally, physically and emotionally – a fatigue I had never ever experienced in my life.

Even five days of a Les Mills Boot Camp instructor training, consisting of 14-hour days, being pushed beyond every physical and mental limit I thought possible, sleep deprivation, body and soul demands, followed by six days of a New Zealand National Hockey tournament with an infected knee, had NOTHING on this. I was totally, and absolutely spent from the surgeries, treatment, stage of recovery and the previous year of dis-ease.

I was unable to do my usual things each day, and when I did, the recovery time was far beyond anything I had ever encountered. A half-day outing to the shops took three days of sitting on the couch to recover from. I felt like a true *couch potato*. This was something so foreign to me that it made me bristle on every inch of my skin. I wanted to be me and do what I normally did, cut off the recognition of pain and then play, but I could not.

It had the upper hand – *IT* (the cancer treatment) was dictating to me what I could do in every moment of the day. The rules I now needed to play by were completely foreign, unacceptable and outrageous to me. I did not know how to deal with this. I was ALWAYS able to overcome physical performance challenges. Even when I had bilateral Achilles debridement and both lower legs in plaster, I was back in shape and playing hockey for New Zealand in Canada five months later. But this was a struggle like no other.

It was necessary to confront my struggles. While listening to a broadcast about taking time for life, Cheryl Richardson voiced these impactful words, "I am forced to have a relationship with the unknown". These powerful words resonated with me as I was grappling with a way forward. What form the relationship took I realised was my choice. It could be a relationship of hatred, fear, anger, regret, guilt, shame or any other negative emotion, or it could be one of thriving with a diagnosis. I didn't have to own the cancer or be best friends with it, but I needed to have a mutual respect for the power and impact it could have on me.

My philosophy in life is to share my gifts with as many people as possible. To have a positive impact on the world so people can enjoy fun, laughter, and live their lives to the fullest - even in the tough times. This forced moment of struggle was the perfect time to live up to and implement my philosophy, and practise what I taught.

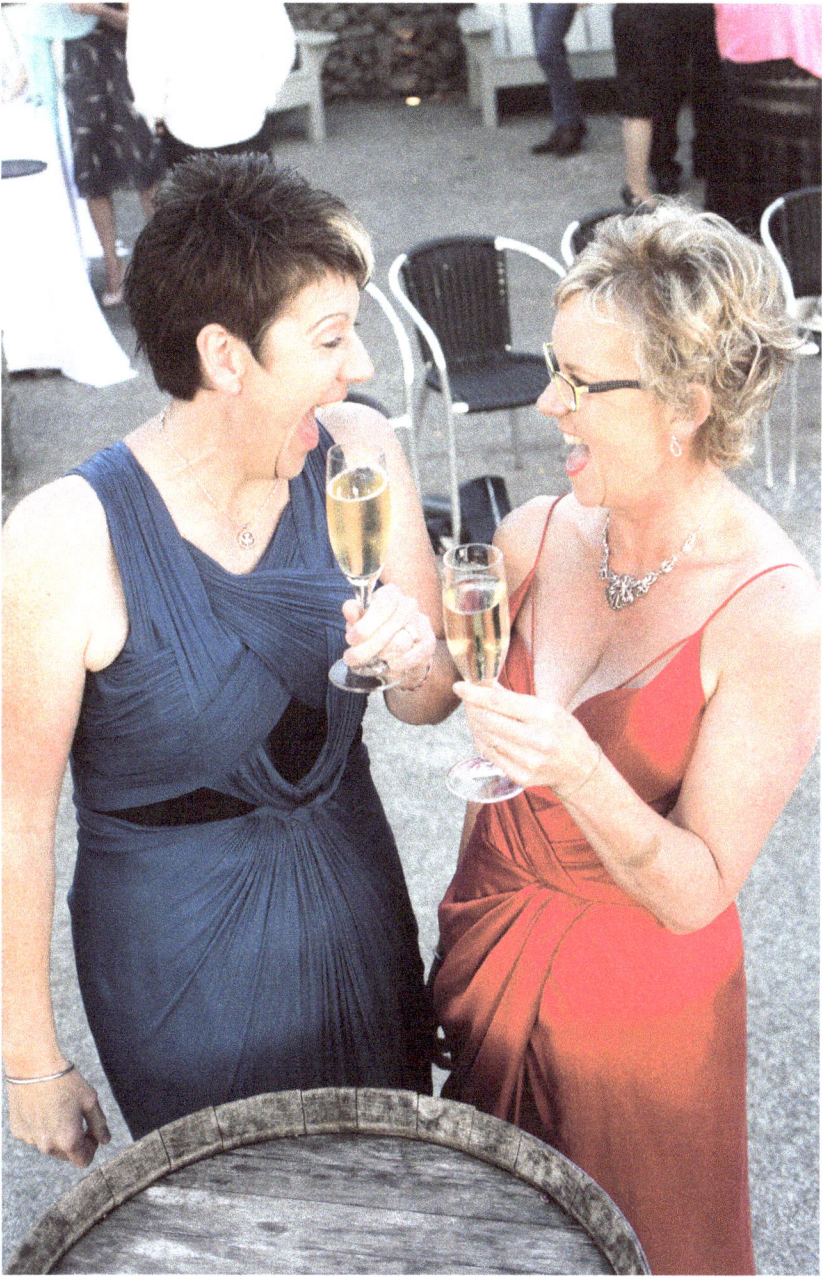

We did it!

Chapter 7

Grit, Willpower and Vulnerability

L earning to push myself outside my comfort zone was something I had done many times before. It requires a mixture of grit, willpower and vulnerability which I knew I had within me. However, this current new challenge was going to test every ounce of these and take these abilities to a whole new level.

Grit is defined as "the tendency to sustain interest in, and effort toward, a very long-term goal" (Von Culin, Tsukayama & Duckworth, 2014, p. 1) and is associated with courage, resilience and hardiness to pursue goals over the long-term with passion and perseverance (Duckworth, Peterson, Matthews & Kelly, 2007).

Grit is more than talent, skills and intellect, all of which I have plenty of, but to get through the challenging times it takes consistent and continuous mental and physical toughness. To activate my grit in that moment, I needed to draw on all my strength, knowledge and passion to persevere, if I was going to get through these next few months at my relative best. I needed the ability to keep going and keep working towards something long-term; never giving up.

Angela Duckworth (US psychologist) explains that people with more *grit* have more self-control mentally, physically and emotionally, which also stops the ascension into catastrophising or an escalation of thoughts assuming the worst will happen (Duckworth, 2016).

An example of activating grit is: "Even though I don't want to engage with people right now, I know that I need to get out of the house as I am becoming very negatively focused". This small step can change the catastrophising thought of "everything is going wrong and I will never be able to get back to work" into something more manageable. This is the first step towards turning an event around.

This is a challenge for us all. Being able to recognise the escalation of thoughts, push the pause button and then do something differently in that moment. The thing that helped me at that time was connecting with inspiring people. I have always loved reading and watching inspiring stories of the underdog who comes out on top, or the person who works extra hard, goes above and beyond and achieves their dream. My favourite is 'Remember the Titans' which displays how a group of stereotypical egos become a tight-knit, high performing team.

This inspires me to keep going, to reach for something better. We all need to recognise our thoughts, language and behaviours, and then purposefully do something to change them when they are barrelling towards the negative. When we show grit, persevere through hard times and achieve our goals despite the setbacks, we are also demonstrating a growth and opportunity mindset.

I realised in that moment, that this was now my time to be that person; the underdog, the person who operates above and beyond, and keeps going no matter what. Life experience has taught me that constructing solutions to unexpected events is no simple matter. We must discover the strengths within and remember previous times of achievement to rise up in the present moment. Now was my time to instigate these characteristics and demonstrate grit and willpower which are effective, regardless of the unfamiliarity or enormity of the situation or event.

Willpower is the ability to resist short-term temptations in order to successfully meet long-term goals. It includes the capacity to 'override' a negative thought, feeling or impulse (Baumeister & Tierney, 2011). Willpower is closely intertwined with self-control and begins with self-awareness. Individuals who are self-aware of their thoughts and feelings have a higher-than-average level of self-control. They engage in making choices that set themselves up to achieve success rather than evoking ongoing challenges.

According to Baumeister and Tierney (2011), the most successful people, defined as happier, healthier and with stronger connections, spend less time struggling with temptations that pull them off track and are therefore more focused. By applying their self-control and willpower to a specific situation, they allow themselves to get the best out of life.

An example of instigating self-control is leaving work on time five days in a row. You set your phone alarm 15 minutes before you choose to leave work to remind you to finish up for the day. You take your mug to the kitchen, rinse it out and recite to yourself, "That's it done for today", and then you leave your work at work. The short-term temptation is to stay and work, the long-term goal is to be healthy and have energy for those at home. Just as muscles are strengthened by regular exercise, consistently exerting self-control improves willpower and strengthens it, over time.

Historical research on self-control is the marshmallow experiment by Mischel and Ebbesen which was completed with 4 to 6-year-olds in 1970. The children were taken one by one into the interview room, given one marshmallow and told if they waited 15 minutes without eating it, they would get another one. One third of the 600 children resisted the temptation and displayed self-control, and therefore willpower. The others gave in, exerted no self-control, and ate the marshmallow. The same children were studied later in life with incredible long-term results. The ones who exhibited higher levels of self-control achieved better at school, had a fulfilling career and were physically healthier. WILLPOWER IS VITAL!

Willpower can also 'run out'. This is because willpower is boosted by our chemical levels of glucose. If we are learning new skills under large amounts of pressure, working outside of our peak energy times, and haven't fuelled our body with healthy foods or liquids, then we will deplete our ability to exert self-control and our willpower WILL run out. If we have not cultivated willpower by increasing our self-awareness and recognising when we need to adjust things (self-control), we become depleted and RUN OUT OF STEAM to make healthy choices (Vonasch, Vohs, Pocheptsova, & Baumeister, 2018).

Engaging in negative self-talk also depletes willpower, lowers the quality of decision making and results in lower performance. When we are thinking and talking negatively our cortisol levels increase, spiralling our emotions downwards, increasing stress, limiting our thoughts, and decreasing the possibilities or opportunities that we perceive are available to us.

An interesting fact is that there are more negative emotional words in the English dictionary than positive (Cacioppo, Gardner, & Berntson, 1997). It's true, and with the higher ratio of negative to positive, comes a propensity to overuse this language which reinforces our negative perspective even more. When we use negative words and thoughts, we create a chemical release in our brain that floods our body and gets interpreted as negative emotions.

When we have sufficient self-awareness to recognise our negative emotions, and enough self-control to deal with them effectively, we spend less time struggling with crises. People with low willpower spend all of what they have to get them out of crises, whereas people with high willpower engage this to *avoid* crises (Baumeister & Tierney, 2011). When we turn all this around to think and talk positive, hopeful, optimistic, and joyful thoughts, we create uplifting emotional and physiological responses in our bodies (Seligman, 2011).

Alex Korb neuroscientist and author states, that when we experience uplifting responses, we produce the chemical serotonin in our bodies which is known as the molecule of willpower (Korb, 2015). Serotonin is also considered to be the natural mood stabiliser and confidence booster. More confidence leads to better decision making and more willpower and individuals with greater willpower are better able to manage stress, deal with conflict and overcome adversity.

Once I had begun to master my willpower to set myself up each day with this optimistic mindset, regardless of how I was feeling, I learned that I needed to also open up to others. I needed to be vulnerable, ask for help, let people know how I was truly coping (or not) on the day. This requires a high degree of being present; enlisting all of my senses in the moment. I am good at this. I learned this from my hockey days, when a ball would come hurtling towards me from a penalty stroke, I had to be fully present with every sense heightened. I needed to bring this skill of being present and integrate it with open, honest, vulnerability, to get amazing things happening.

Vulnerability is also a part of initiating self-awareness and willpower. Opening up and being vulnerable to hear the reactions of others can certainly be scary. By stating, "I have just been diagnosed with cancer" to others is displaying vulnerability. By saying, "I don't have the energy to do this today", is vulnerability. By asking "can you help me do this" is vulnerability.

As Brené Brown (Professor and researcher of courage, shame and vulnerability) describes; *"vulnerability is not winning or losing; it's having the courage to show up and be seen when we have no control over the outcome. Vulnerability is not weakness; it's our greatest measure of courage"* (2015, p. 4). I had to learn this the hard way. It was not something I previously had in my toolkit, but I'm so glad I put myself out there and chose those moments to be vulnerable.

It is important to embrace the feeling of vulnerability within uncontrollable moments, and to express any shame and guilt we may feel. In my case, I felt shame that I had let myself down, that I had let others down, and that my body had failed to support my health. For me, the guilt was around not performing at my best and causing a problem for others.

When we recognise and admit to ourselves when we are being vulnerable, we allow our inner wisdom and knowing to shine through and be heard. Inner wisdom is like the advice we would share with a dear friend; the loving encouragement we give to ourselves to push the limits and reach new heights, but often fail to listen to. Listening to and acting upon the advice from our inner wisdom is incredibly empowering, even though at first scary. This is not about being selfish or seeking attention, this is about acceptance of our own situation and what we require in the moment.

When we display vulnerability to others, we open ourselves up to higher levels of self-awareness which allows us to engage in higher levels of willpower. They are all interconnected. Self-awareness of what is needed in that moment. Willpower to take charge of the moment, work through the adversity and create a path forward. With the integration of grit, willpower and vulnerability we KNOW that we can make anything happen and we have the abilities and skills to be resilient.

To instigate my triad of grit, willpower and vulnerability, I drew on the lessons I had learned from challenging experiences across all of my life, whether these had been successes, failures, mistakes, or achievements. There is always a lesson to be learned if we are open to it.

Like when Dad told me that he only had a very short time to live in 2008. He was showing me around the hospice (while I pushed him in a wheelchair), chatting and laughing with the staff and patients. People who had become an important part of his life. I was totally *present*. I was right there with him every step of the way. The smells, the sights and the sounds of people making the most of every single day they had remaining. Regardless of the lack of control I felt inside, I engaged with all of my senses at that specific time.

Dad seemed to be in good heart, despite his diagnoses of leukaemia in 1997, prostate cancer in 2004, and lymphoma in 2007. During this time, he also had a hip fracture and an infected big toe that required amputation. Being present to hear his laughter, his jokes, have meaningful conversations with many of the people in the unit, and to feel their realness, honesty and vulnerability, allowed me to believe that there is always a reason to be grateful. That was actually the last time he was conscious and interacting with them all. After a short and abrupt decline, he passed away on the 23rd November, 2008. As hard as it was to be in that moment, I would not have missed that moment with him for anything.

Another experience that I drew on was receiving a phone call from the Intensive Care Unit at Palmerston North Hospital on the evening of 7th June, 2011. The Emergency Department nurse told me that I needed to get there urgently. It was Mum. This entailed a rapid trip from Wellington to Palmerston North (2 hours) to see Mum after an acute ambulance admission. They did not think she would last the night.

Having this news thrown at me was like being hit by a bus (or what I would imagine that to feel like). It was my turn to be there for Mum and support her, as she had been there for me so many times throughout my life. This was not a time for me to become caught up in my own fears, worries, or concerns about the small details or misfortunes in life. This was friggin' real. My Mum and BEST FRIEND was in intensive care on a CPAP machine (a forced surrogate breathing machine), fighting for her life. I needed to be there for her and not be distracted by me.

My ability to recognise my emotions and leave the unnecessary behind, to be serious, vulnerable, real, and ask the tough questions of the medical staff, was needed in this moment. My Mum passed away on the third day – 9th June, 2011. I mustered my grit and determination once again, stepped up and did what I needed to do.

No matter what life has thrown at me, the good, the bad and the ugly, I have learned that there is ALWAYS more in my tank. At those times when we feel mentally, physically, and emotionally spent, there is always more! Knowing and experiencing that my tank (my whole *self*) is bigger, deeper, and has more fuel and resilience than I could ever imagine, has been one of the strongest attributes to get me through the initial stages of my new uncontrollable moment.

The human body in all its wonder can deal and cope with all sorts of amazing pressures that are way beyond our wildest dreams. The possibilities are limitless. We often limit ourselves by thinking we are at the end of our rope, and cannot give or do anymore, but there is always more in our tank. We only know this and experience this when we get out of our comfort zone.

I've had many experiences in life which forced me outside of my comfort zone, but I instigated strategies and learned to thrive and not just survive. This gave me confirmation that I could indeed deal with the unknown.

I vividly remember an incident during a hockey game that required me to step out of my comfort zone and into the unknown. I was standing in my goal circle on the hockey turf three minutes away from winning the New Zealand National Hockey Championships. I was ready for anything, although physically drained and hurting, and breathing heavily with huge amounts of adrenaline surging through my body. This was a moment of immense nervousness with both familiar and unfamiliar components.

It was time to focus on the important tasks in that situation and tune out anything that was going to distract me or deplete my willpower. It was time to be totally *in the zone*. I narrowed my focus into the present moment and kept watching, listening, and directing my team where I needed them to be. Engaging mentally and physically in every play of the game so I could perform at the required exceptional level.

The crowd was cheering so loudly we could hardly hear each other calling directions on the turf. As the seconds ticked away we were one step closer to being National Champions. The best team in the whole country! The pressure was immense. The emotions were almost brimming over but needed to be kept in check. Right up until the last whistle we had to focus and control everything we possibly could – our game plan, our skills, our defence, our communication with each other, and most importantly we needed to work together.

We became the National Champions. It was our turn to celebrate and boy we did! We all grouped together jumping up and down, yelling and screaming, hugging each other with the hugest of smiles enjoying our win. Even though the unfamiliarity of this amount of pressure was scary, our willpower got us through. Making calculated decisions, pushing ourselves beyond our self-limiting beliefs, and just doing it. We succeeded.

Life is a team effort. We cannot go through life or adversity on our own. We need the collective support of at least one other person. Humans are wired for connection and in times of challenge, this is even more acute. Creating and maintaining strong connections with our team mates, our family or our friends is vital and requires us to be vulnerable.

To live a happy and healthy life takes courage, "*showing up as our true self and being seen*" (Brown, 2015, p. 4). When we say, ("insert your own uncontrollable moment") has just happened, we give ourselves permission to react, feel, yell, or even cry. Accepting the situation *as-is* and feeling all the emotions that are part of the experience. These may include anger, fear, disbelief, shame, guilt, relief, anxiety or betrayal.

If we continue to respond negatively we may become sicker, take longer to recover, or end up in a dark place mentally. The words we use have a significant impact on our emotions. (More about this in chapter 8).

I am a total believer in saying the word 'cancer', as it helped me to take control and lessen the extreme negative stigma and power the word can bring with it. I know for others this might not be the case. They refer to cancer as 'The Big C', or are not even able to label it. For me, it was important to say the word because it took the sting out of it, and let me control what I could.

I also chose not to use the words *fight* or *battle,* as these stir up all sorts of negative, combative feelings and words. When we invest our thoughts and energy into negative words or events we cannot control, then this depletes our willpower and induces high levels of negative chemicals to be released throughout the body. Our emotions and physiological reactions align themselves with this negative response.

Whereas when we choose to engage in positive thoughts, words, moments of joy and openness, we reduce stress and tension mentally, physically and emotionally. When we recognise the situation *as-is* with grit, willpower and vulnerability, we are better able to handle the challenging situations. I was *forced* to have a relationship with the uncontrollable moment and I purposefully chose a positive, optimistic and meaningful response. What will you choose?

Your limitless possibilities!

1) Create new positive routines
   - Connect with and repeat the new routines as being your *new normal*
   - Develop consistent routines that bring out the best in you
2) See the humour in things
   - Watch funny movies, laugh with people, read funny stories
3) Choose positive language
   - Be conscious of your thoughts, self-talk and language
   - Be involved in activities you love doing
   - Find the *flow* in what you do
4) Be present - begin simple mindfulness (active mindful moments within activities like walking, cleaning teeth, or during more traditional times of meditation)
5) *Three good things* and why – do this every day and in those moments when you are feeling down or blue
6) Instigate a daily practice of stillness – my space/time immersed in the moment, say to yourself, "All I hear and see is exactly what is front of me"

Section Three

COUNTERACTING THE VERDICT

* * *

Affirmation: "I control the controllables and re-ignite my power"

Chapter 8

Powerless Negotiation

After seven days since being given the diagnosis over the phone, I received no new information, no plan, and still no solution. I felt powerless in my quest to find a way forward. This whole uncontrollable moment of being given a cancer diagnosis and proceeding moments during this week, drove me crazy.

My first hospital appointment started with the baby doctor (she seemed like she was 12 years old but of course she wasn't, she was a doctor in training). She repeated exactly what I had been told over the phone, "We need to do more tests, scans and speak with the Oncology doctor to confirm a treatment plan".

On the inside I was fuming, I already knew this and needed more information, but she gave me nothing. I wanted to scream and yell. I felt powerless. Elizabeth and I kept asking questions; we needed answers. The baby doctor was doing her best to follow the rules. We wanted to break all those rules and get the answers then. I was scared and freaking out. In my eyes that baby doctor knew more than she was letting on, and I was going to get those answers no matter what.

Both Elizabeth and I pushed for more information again, but it didn't make any difference. We asked to see the baby doctor's senior to find out more. She arrived but that didn't change the situation for us either. The frustration levels were rising in that room and not in a positive way. We were wanting information to answer the unknown.

Desperation was escalating and we were not getting what we wanted or needed. The thoughts in my head were racing. The dialogue in my head went something like this, "Yes, I understand that I need to wait for the recent surgery to heal before any treatment can start, but I'm a fast healer and I recover quickly. Can't you understand this. I just want this over with".

Apparently, there was a process to follow. But I didn't give a crap about their processes at that point in time. I had just been diagnosed with cancer. I needed answers now. If there was a process to follow, I would find a better way through it. Just like I always do.

We had to reschedule our days and Elizabeth's work times to attend the Oncology outpatient visits and this was all we were told. There was no choice of appointment times and very little notice was given. I felt really bad for Elizabeth, as the first face-to-face conversation with the medical team about this whole new crazy situation was everything I had already told her. We had no further information. I kept thinking to myself, Elizabeth deserves to know more, she needs to know how this game will play out. I could sort myself out and cope in my usual way, but she was sitting on the side-line with even less control than I had. And that was next to none!

Unbeknown to us, procedures were ticking along in the background including histopathology, cytology and genetic testing; specialists and surgeons weaving their magic, discussing my case, with all of them working together to design the best way forward for me. I was not the only person they were seeing with a cancer diagnosis of course, so there were limited machines (PET, CT, Radiotherapy) that could be used, limited staff available, and they were actually following protocols that had a great deal of evidence behind them. But I didn't know this.

At that time, I cared little for their justification – "you just need to wait and heal first". I wanted answers, and I wanted them now. I needed a way forward and a solution to take the edge off my fear BUT this was their turf and I had to play their game.

Finally, the phone calls for appointments came thick and fast. Every time the phone rang with 'private number' flashing up on the screen, my heart would skip a beat, and still does. It would be another person from the medical team scheduling or rescheduling an appointment. It was a constant reminder that I was now part of a team I never thought I would be part of.

When I was given an appointment time, I had to take it. There was no choice of an alternative unless I wanted to wait another two or three months then yes, I could pick and choose any time I wanted. My power to choose how this game played out had been removed. But if I wanted answers, results and action as soon as possible, then I had to take the appointment I was given. I was shit scared and being a newbie to this game I had to toe the line. I had to conform to their rules. There were no options and it was no longer my choice. I wanted to have all the appointments, medical visits and tests happening as fast as possible, so I would always say yes. This contributed to the feeling of being at *their* beck and call. It was a catch 22 situation.

No day was mine anymore. Appointment after appointment after appointment with strangers were how my days played out. To make matters worse this game was being played in the side of the hospital that no-one wants to go near, the Cancer Centre. I had to be vulnerable once again, and allow these strangers into my life when they wanted, not when I was ready or able. I was in the midst of turmoil, coming to grips with a diagnosis that looked like doomsday, and I felt like everything was being taken away from me. My health, my independence, my vibrant energy, and my ability to bounce forward had been crushed.

People were telling me what to do, when to do it, and how to do it. I wasn't able to do a great deal for myself and I had become reliant on others. This was totally against my usual way of life. My body was not recovering as fast as usual due to a year of being extremely depleted. I had put on a mask and hidden the extent of my dis-ease for most of that time, however I couldn't fool my body. It was abnormally out of balance and my health was deteriorating rapidly.

During the previous four months I had received an emergency iron infusion, copious amounts of chemicals and medications, undergone two surgical procedures, and been dealt a diagnosis that had sent my entire body into severe trauma. All the while I was mentally and emotionally exhausted from a work environment that had become toxic, from the higher management levels down to the teams. Here I was, a strong, powerful, independent woman, precipitously deteriorating mentally, physically, and emotionally feeling absolutely useless. I had become POWERLESS.

I was powerless in my diagnosis and treatment regime. The medical team had full control over who, what, when, where and how. They were the experts in the treatment of the cancer and I allowed them to take over the decision making. It wasn't about ME as a person, it was about the symptoms, the diagnosis and the pre-determined treatment plan. I was just a number, a name that popped up on a file, part of their system, just another task in the day.

There were many occasions when I felt de-personalised. They didn't know me and they didn't know who I was or what I was capable of. I am me because of the strength of my heritage, my family, my experiences, my values, morals, and beliefs, yet this wasn't acknowledged. It was like I had regressed and become a child again, being told what to do and how my life would unfold. Here I was over 40 and yet I had lost control of my own life.

Most of the people I was dealing with were much younger than me; this was such a role reversal. I needed to trust the youngsters and their skills and abilities, but I had the expertise of who I was, how to get the best out of my body, and how to bounce forward from adversity. Regardless of my abilities, throughout radiotherapy my timetable was determined each day by them.

The medical staff told me that the side effects would get worse as the weeks of treatment continued. The Oncology nurse warned me about what would happen week by week. It was alarming. I wasn't sure what was worse; the diagnosis or the side effects of the treatment. As the weeks went on the side effects escalated and continued to accumulate even after the treatment ended. They were right when they said the worst could be expected three to four weeks after treatment.

My weekly check-ups at the Oncology clinic were punctuated with the comment, "Oh it'll get much worse". I was fearing for my life in terms of the cancer diagnosis and if that wasn't enough, I needed to expect to suffer terribly from the treatment and its side effects. I remember chatting with a fellow team mate as we were waiting for radiotherapy, and he had been warned with absolute conviction as well that his health would be compromised in so many ways due to the treatment. This made no sense to me. How could this get any worse than I was already feeling? I was usually so good at sorting things out, why couldn't I sort this?

As I began to realise that I was feeling out of control and losing my grip on the game plan, it was time to work out how I could have moments of being ME in this situation. I got that the process needed to follow a specific system, but I am a person with a name. I have a story, and strengths, and I love people. I wanted to keep living and give my all to every part of this game of life. They didn't want to know about me or my story. The questions and discussions were about signs and symptoms, always referring back to the diagnosis. It wasn't about ME as a person.

This was totally against my usual way of working and functioning so it was sending me into a spin. This was something that was life threatening, and traditional stigma around cancer is often one of fear, devastation and isolation. I wanted none of this. I decided to take on the challenge to get to know these experts, have them in my corner and take my power back within the realms of possibility.

I was powerless at home, still recovering from the surgery. In the beginning of my recovery I was totally reliant on Elizabeth for everything. From getting assistance with showering, dressing, and moving about the house, to needing food and drink left out during the day for nourishment (due to the weight of containers and equipment). I was unable to leave home, drive or catch public transport. I needed to ask for help. One day I even managed to get myself stuck while reaching into the fridge for a small jar of jam. I didn't have the ability to engage my core (midsection) to stand back up, so here I was half in and half out of the fridge at a ridiculous angle with nowhere to go. Again, I needed to call for help.

Prior to this recovery time, I was also powerless at work. An environment where trust did not occur and we were not supported to excel at all. There was no way I could change an entire departmental culture that was unwilling to grow. In the hierarchy of that system I was placed at the bottom. If I was going to influence any change I needed energy and lots of it, but this wasn't going to happen. I had decided I needed to leave, it was just a matter of when.

There was a culture of mistrust, disrespect and poor communication throughout the department. This made forming any kind of team connection extremely challenging. Micro-managing had become the way to stifle any individual creativity or initiative. The ability to make individual decisions had long been stripped away. There was an underlying belief that more hours in the office meant more work, regardless of effectiveness. It was like the clock had been wound back and we were in the 'workhouse' days. Moments of happiness, laughter or joy were frowned upon. It was not a happy place to be.

I was unable to keep pushing myself when I needed the energy elsewhere. Even though I was wearing my 'skidlid' (goalkeeper helmet) to deflect the absurdities of working in a toxic environment, it was not prevailing. I had donned the 'mask' to protect myself from the negativity and stay above the destructive nature of the environment. I had also stopped listening to my body, a skill I had learnt at hockey that served me well to stay at the top of my game.

As a lecturer, I was committed to this game and intent on being there for the students until the end of the year. What I realised later during my recovery was that as my mask became more remarkable, the environment and people caused more harmful effects on me mentally, physically and emotionally. I needed to be jolted into action. If I was not going to make the decision to leave, then something bigger than me was going to make this happen.

For several months, Elizabeth and a number of friends had been telling me to leave the role. But in my mind I saw this as buckling to the pressure and giving in. I do not surrender! If you were on my hockey turf and I was in goal, my motto was "never allow both the ball and the person to get past me". I would give it everything to prevent a goal against my team. I saw surrender as weakness and failure, and in this instance I would not give in either.

In hindsight I now know that I was denying myself the real truth. The irrational story I was telling myself was that I would be letting the students down if I left before the end of the year, when in fact the only person I was letting down was myself. The cost of believing this irrational story was my health. There were a number of warning signs but I was too proud to see them. Too proud to admit I needed to ease up, get help or even stop all together. I personally believe that things happen for a reason and the diagnosis was one of them.

As hard as it was to fly the white flag and walk away from the situation, I needed to call it quits. I desperately wanted to help turn the workplace around as I knew I had the skills to do so, but no-one was listening. I had to finally admit that this was one game I would never win, walk away and focus on other things. I handed in my resignation, copped more flack, but walked away with my head held high.

I am a believer in the fact that our environment contributes to our health – this incorporates the physical, emotional and spiritual environments around us. When one of these things is out of kilter, it has a huge impact on the others. This in turn will eventually show up as a health problem. Our body will always win! If we push ourselves to exhaustion without noticing the warning signs, our bodies will react and break down in some way e.g. migraine, stomach ulcers, heart problems, or even a fracture.

Our body will find a way to stop us because we are not stopping ourselves and changing things to promote flourishing health. If a situation or relationship is ongoing and predominately negative, we know this will activate harmful hormones and chemicals, and eventually cause cellular breakdown.

Dr Bruce Lipton, a developmental cell biologist, stated that he finally understood the key to life after many years of scientific experiment, "It's in the environment, stupid" (Lipton, 2005, p22). He describes how the external environment (e.g. the air quality, temperature, noise levels) impacts the internal human environment (our cells, tissues and organs).

If the quality of the environment is contaminated in any way, we will also be affected.

He first showed this in a culture dish, where cells physically moved away from toxins that were introduced to the environment. If they didn't move away, there was a cessation or stunting of cell growth which is known as 'faltering effects'. Lipton also explored how a healthy environment invigorated cells to thrive, yet when the environment was less than optimal, the cells faltered. When he re-adjusted the environment, he showed that the 'sick' cells were revitalised. Cells can be regenerated with the right remediation, but this is dependent on the amount of damage already experienced.

Lipton states that just like the cells in the culture dish, we are shaped by our environment – both physical and energetic. If the people around us are demeaning, dismissive or constantly disagreeable, this will affect us on a cellular level. If they live their life with a negative approach and we are around this all the time, it will eventually stunt the development and ongoing growth of our body's cells.

He identified that the signals and energetic messages emanating from positive or negative thoughts are the key to whether a human thrives or falters. Humans are immersed in their environment and any fluctuations can have drastic effects on their mental, physiological, and emotional health (Lipton, 2005).

The natural behaviours of cells and humans is either to retreat and protect oneself (from danger and toxins) or move towards something that supports health and life. However, humans can choose to gravitate towards conditions that nourish and assist in growth, move away from threats as a protective behaviour, or stay in a negative environment where we will eventually die.

Included in the environment of our cells are our beliefs. Beliefs act like a filter on a camera, always changing and focusing on how we see the world. Lipton highlights that our cellular biology adapts to those beliefs. For example, if we believe that we don't deserve to have good experiences or positive relationships, then we might stay in an abusive relationship rather than move out of it. This will increase the stress levels experienced in our body and ultimately change the cellular structures, which in turn can cause chronic physical and mental illness.

When we recognise the power that our beliefs have on our biology, we have identified a vital factor for a healthier lifestyle. While we cannot change the codes of our genetic makeup, we can change our thoughts, our beliefs and our environment. Lipton has proven that it is not gene-directed hormones and neurotransmitters that control us, but our beliefs and environment that control the body and mind, and therefore our lives (2005).

One of the many learnings about cells and molecular structures of the body I embraced during this time is the effect of the human consciousness on water molecules. Dr Emoto, a Japanese researcher, identified the huge impact that words have on the molecular structure of water (2007). He first viewed water molecules from mountains, rivers and underground springs through a microscope and identified normal types of structures. He then exposed the water vials to negative or positive environments and words.

The negative environment included heavy metal music, negative words being said directly to the water, and negative messages written on the vials. The effect was astounding when re-viewed. The molecules had distorted into ugly crystalline formations. When he exposed the vials to a positive environment of classical music, positive spoken and written affirmations, the molecules formed beautifully shaped crystals resembling intricate snowflakes. Same water, different environment, different outcomes.

This had me thinking about my thoughts and the self-talk that I

CHRISTINE BURNS

used. If the human body is approximately 60 – 75% water, then the words I hear and say would impact the molecular structure inside my body. If I am thinking and talking in a negative or disempowering way, this would be harmful to both cells and body structures, and negatively influence my recovery.

I started to recognise the direct impact my attitude, thoughts and words could have on my body, and realised I needed to adjust my 'top six inches' (thought processes) and trigger my optimistic approach. If I was to turn this diagnosis around and begin thinking in a more positive and optimistic light, then this would compel my body to heal with power and energy.

Suzanne Segerstrom, a Psychology Professor at the University of Kentucky (known for her research in optimism), defines optimism as "generalised positive expectations for the future" (2005, p 195). She elucidates how optimism is an attitude which can influence our mood and our environment. Research has revealed that humans prefer to interact with positive and optimistic people rather than negative, pessimistic ones (Segerstrom, 2011). Positive people have an energy we enjoy and are naturally drawn to, even when we are not aware of it. In contrast, if a person is in a bad, grumpy or negative mood, they are more likely to be avoided.

Exuding optimism is still something that will occur during adverse situations for the optimistic person. This ability empowers optimistic people to withstand a great deal of negativity and pressure, often unbeknown to their friends, colleagues or those around them (Seligman, 2011).

The longer an individual remains in a negative environment, the deeper the effects, mentally, physically and emotionally. When the human body is subjected to these negative environments for a long period of time it will become unbalanced. When the body is out of balance it responds with a number of warning signals. These warning signals may include headaches, lack of concentration, irritable moods, or mental fatigue. When stress is chronic, the body responds by suppressing the immune system, interrupting digestion, interfering with sleep patterns, and hindering the reproductive system.

I had endometriosis for many years which resulted in surgeries in my 20's and further major surgery in my 30's. During the year of being in a toxic work environment in 2015/2016, the endometriosis intensified in severity. Things became worse, much worse. The pain increased tenfold, an excessive amount of bleeding was happening almost daily, lower back pain was extreme, and my iron levels were plummeting.

A research team from the University of British Columbia and Johns Hopkins Medicine (Anglesio, 2017) identified that endometriosis could occur due to mutations in endometrial cells. While a DNA (genetic molecule) mutation is necessary to initiate cancer, scientists have observed that stress appears to speed up the development of cancerous tumours (Krantz et al., 2011). I guess when one mutant cell changes the trajectory of health in a very short time, the cells become powerful and can cause us to lose perspective. If I had only taken a peep out from under my mask I would have seen the many warning signals.

At that stage and throughout the time of illness, diagnosis and treatment, I felt my power constantly being eroded. So, what is power and why is it necessary? I define power in this instance as self-belief and ownership of who you are – your authentic self with your opinions, values, views, needs and desires.

Power is not about egotistical, authoritative, or overbearing behaviour. It is not about having control over others. Personal power is a state of mind. An attitude where you take responsibility for your own decisions and actions, and have the ability to protect yourself from the negative influences of others. It is about standing up for your values, being confident in who you are, and contributing to the world around you in a positive and effective way.

Realising that these feelings of powerlessness were not assisting my recovery from surgery, or setting me up to be at my best throughout treatment, I needed to change what I was thinking and doing. I had to become responsible for my thoughts again. The one thing in my power at that moment was that I could choose my thoughts. I am the rightful owner of what goes through my 'top six inches'; no one else gets to decide that.

I knew that thoughts created feelings (emotions) which lead to actions. If I wanted to change the way I felt about the situation and influence my cells to thrive, then I needed to change the thoughts that were running through my head. If it was up to me to manage my emotions, then it was crucial to gain control over the parts that I could control and recapture my self-belief.

Chapter 9

Solitary Confinement

During the first month after diagnosis, my mind would go on a journey of negative and terrifying options and finish with a worst-case scenario all by itself by the end of the day. This worrying journey would make everything worse. I would lie in bed confined in my solitude and just think to myself, "I don't want to die, this is not my time". In the early stages after diagnosis, the moments I had on my own in silence were the toughest. My mind would begin to conjure up all kinds of unpleasant and undesirable outcomes.

The story in these moments would rise up and go something like this… "This cannot be happening; I would leave behind the person I love most in the world. My family would be without a sister, an aunty, a great aunty. The people I had met, influenced, impacted and had interactions with, would remember me as 'the one that was', the person they used to know, the person who wasn't here anymore. Then I would be just a distant memory.

This isn't the life I had planned. How could I have such amazing relationships with people, super-amazing plans to empower people to be their true authentic selves and follow their passions, be one of the chosen ones to change the world, and then this happens? Why is it that I have committed to the person I love most and within one year I end up like this?"

Sometimes my pillow case would be soaked with my tears as they fell silently each night. I was scared for myself and I was scared for Elizabeth. If I said nothing and kept quiet then I wouldn't worry her. In fact, if I did not tell anyone, then maybe the dream would go away. But it wasn't a dream - it was real. At times I felt confused, disheartened and disconnected. Throughout the day I would have moments of feeling relatively healthy and then it was like being on death's door (or what I felt like death's door might be).

Treatment for me was more often in the morning. I'd be the healthy-looking one walking into the dark, dreary waiting room for the cancer patients, smiling and laughing. I would be called through for radiation treatment, immobilised under the giant transformer, left in the room on my own, and then the transformer would buzz and whirr around me working its magic.

Every Wednesday after treatment was check-up time with the Radiation Oncologist in the Cancer Centre. This was the day I'd be reminded in no uncertain terms that I was part of a group of people who had received a death threat, where life had become temperamental. I was reminded of my impermanence and no matter where I looked I saw the word *cancer*. There were no smiling faces, except mine and Elizabeth's. The vibe was depressing and many people assumed the role of helpless patient.

I would sway back and forth in my perception that I was healthy and doing well, to the cancer patient dodging side effects, to feeling ill and just like everyone else in that specific area of the hospital. I'd have a laugh with Elizabeth in the waiting room, chat with others, and be present in the moment. Then just as I would feel my energy starting to rise, the Radiation Oncologist would ask how the side effects were impacting me, remind me of where I was up to in my treatment and describe how the next phase would destroy more cells (healthy and unhealthy).

And then out would come their repeated statement of, "Oh it will get much worse". Then I'd have to sit and wait to see the next person in hospital. Sometimes I'd sit and wait for what seemed like a lifetime, and other times not. The waiting, the unknown, was unsettling.

To leave behind the impact of treatment for the day, being in hospital and the negative reminders of what was happening, we would go to a café and enjoy a strong, skinny piccolo. This routine would ground me and helped me gain a sense of control back into my day. Elizabeth and I would debrief on what had happened, talk about anything negative or positive that may have come up during the visit, and then slowly readjust into how the day was panning out.

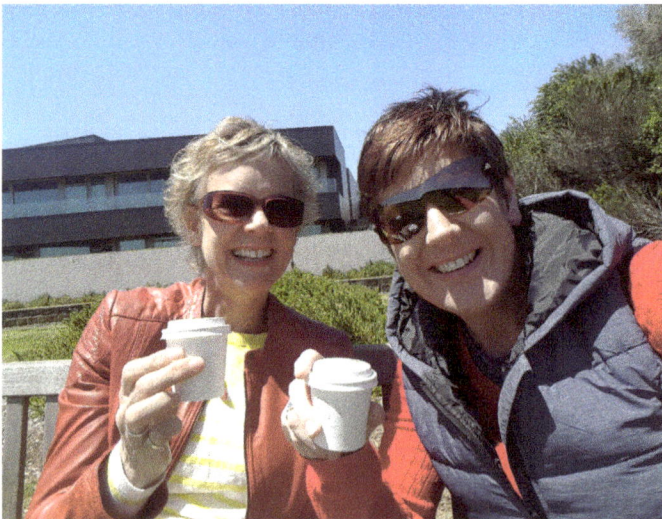

The after treatment coffee ritual and celebration

CHRISTINE BURNS

On the odd occasion when I was on my own for these sessions I'd enjoy my piccolo coffee and read an inspiring magazine or book (when my post-treatment buzzing head would allow me). In the café I'd look like any other regular in there. Tidily dressed, make-up on, smiling, and talking with the people in the café. I would have more than the average number of trips to the bathroom than most people in the café, due to the stimulation from treatment. Sometimes I'd even have two coffees because it tasted so good.

Elizabeth would head off to work and I'd go home for a rest, do some chores, a little bit of work on our business, and sometimes even have a sleep. My ears would ring, I'd feel fidgety and on edge from the treatment, and then work out what food might stay in my body that day. If I was feeling really good (this is relative!) I'd go for a bike ride to the beach, which is about a 7km roundtrip.

Noticing the moments I felt good was when I would 'fill up my cup'. This is when I would purposefully engage and savour the moments. I *knew* these were the moments that would help me recover, heal and shift my head space (even for a short moment in time) to a place where I could see a future of health and happiness. It gave me a little more energy, enhanced my positive thoughts, and increased the 'happy chemicals' in my body. I would notice my body feeling like a healthier machine, and my head would quieten down.

There were often moments when the life and death questions ran riot in my head. The reality of this situation was still intensifying and the doom and gloom associated with a cancer diagnosis was mounting. Was the treatment doing what it was meant to? Would I be here for a short time or a long time? What else could I do to strengthen my chances of making sure everything was working the way it needed to? What could I do to take back some control of all the madness?

There was what seemed like an animal instinct emerge in me. When you see a sick animal remove itself from its peer group, family and community, you know something is wrong. It's exactly how I saw myself. I thought that if I removed myself from others then I would conserve my energy. Then with no-one else around I could do what I needed to do without distraction, and this would limit the negative impact I had on others so they could be themselves and not be scared for me. These thoughts and actions were real for me at the time; they made sense for where my head was at.

To cope with the anxious feelings of the unknown I went deeper into my solitude where I felt confined and even 'locked down'. It was a strategy I used to protect myself, cope mentally and emotionally, and preserve energy. Going into isolation was my reaction to the situation.

I knew in the past when I needed to perform at my best I would hunker down, separate myself from the hype, and focus on what I needed to do to achieve the best possible outcome. However, these times of lockdown were in relation to achieving at sport, achieving in my role as a lecturer, team leader, or delivering the best performance I could. I had never been in this exact situation before. I felt threatened by something I did not know and could not control. It all seemed way bigger than me.

Adding to my perception of isolation was the feeling that many people I had once seen as friends, allies, supporters, or people I could rely on when the chips were down, were finding the whole situation really tough. I felt at times like some of these people had abandoned me. Maybe they didn't know what to say or do, or they felt scared, so they stayed away. Many people stopped all communication with Elizabeth and myself and generally slipped out of the picture.

I guess in a way this was their own form of 'lockdown', to protect and preserve themselves from embarrassment or awkwardness so they could process the situation from their own point of view. I found the lack of contact, or general support for Elizabeth or me, hard to figure out. At times it angered me when people didn't reply, get in touch or check-in, as it made me feel unworthy. There were times when I thought to myself, "Do you not get how big or bad this is for me? I've had a diagnosis thrown at me and you are healthy, so help me out. If it was the other way around I would contact you, I would check-in with you".

There were moments my performance-driven mindset worked against me too. When I began to open up and admit that I wasn't my usual self to others, it didn't evoke the outcome I expected. When I said I was at 85% of my usual that was bad for me. However, my ability to cope and deal with adversity is rather high, so I appeared to be doing quite well in many people's eyes. Interpretation certainly worked against me during those times.

It wasn't all bad on the support, friendship, or assistance side of things. I must say some people were absolutely amazing. There were people I hadn't had a great deal of contact with for a while who jumped up and helped out with encouragement, support, gifts, financial assistance, time, energy and love. For that I am truly grateful.

Initially I didn't want to tell people I had been diagnosed with cancer. I believed that as soon as I said the 'C' word people would push me aside and treat me like a leper, or as if I was going to drop dead in front of them. In my head, telling people about the diagnosis would cause them to put me into the 'sick box' and that was not something I wanted.

At first this was my own way of dealing with the situation. I knew it was real but somehow if I didn't talk a great deal about it, and pretended to be my normal self around people I knew, then maybe I could cope better. After a while, I realised I wasn't coping, I wasn't happy and I knew something had to change, but I didn't know what.

I worked out why the disconnection got to me so much. It went against my values of compassion, kindness and helping people out. If I couldn't find the support and strength from others outside of me then I would lock down and go inwards to find the strength and sustenance.

There is such a negative take on cancer in society these days. It is much better than it used to be, and there is now a light at the end of the tunnel for many people who receive a cancer diagnosis. However, it is harrowing to be in that alarming moment of being told you have it.

The usual deal is to think: Cancer = Death.

I was fully aware of research that identified how a positive, healthy mindset could increase health outcomes. This compelled me to draft my initial (warped) plan. It went like this: To get the support I needed, and for people to be at their best when interacting with me, I wouldn't tell them anything was wrong.

This ignorance on my part would keep them from treating me differently and therefore I would be 'normal'. Being 'normal' would keep me going as if there was nothing wrong with me. It sounds crazy doesn't it? It took me quite some time to realise in fact that it was crazy and did not elicit help from others.

To be in a place where I could receive from others I needed to connect with my best self and allow my vulnerable, softer and compassionate side to shine. As Mahatma Gandhi and the Dalai Lama identify, for a change in perception and a change in reality to occur the first change must come from within.

"You must be the change you wish to see in the world"
– Mahatma Gandhi –

"First one must change. I first watch myself, check myself, then expect changes from others"
– Dalai Lama –

I expected, wanted, and needed people to show their compassion towards me, and to check in with me. But, how could I expect that from others if I wasn't showing it towards myself first? If I was pretending that I was normal when my world was crashing down around my ears then I was not being honest with myself. Therefore, if I was not being honest with myself, why would anyone else be honest and open with me?

The first step I took to being honest with myself was to go within and work out what I needed at the time. My initial thoughts were to 'lock down' because I didn't want others to treat me like I was going to die. I felt that If I stayed away from people and did what I needed to each day then I could *survive*. When I say lock down I am referring to my own limits and levels of participation in life. There were many people who I interacted with in the hospital system, publicly, and friends who were amazed at what I was doing to make it through.

The second step of being honest with myself was utilising the 'lockdown' periods as a way to conserve physical energy, recharge my soul battery and be present in the moment. This stage of lockdown allowed me to slow down and have a sense of calm, peace and realness of the moment. To experience the toughness, the unknown, the positive fun times and the reality of just *what the hell* was going on.

These intentional lockdown times, were an opportunity for me to reflect on what I was truly thinking. There was no blocking out the hard thoughts or the scary possibilities. Just allowing all of my thoughts to rise up without grabbing hold of any of them, instead acknowledging them, leaving them unchanged, and allowing them to sail on down the river of passing thoughts.

This was hard and let me tell you this. When that thought jumps into your head that you might not be here for much longer, there is a great deal of angst and many other emotions that surge forward. Sitting with these thoughts and emotions swirling around in that river of turmoil was at times like an out-of-control whirlpool. But the longer I sat with these thoughts and feelings, the less the whirlpool drowned me, and the river once again began to flow.

In the self-induced lockdown time I also thought about what my loved ones were going through (as this was not an experience I was going through on my own). I knew I was not alone on the journey.

For me to be the best version of myself, and be mentally and emotionally healthy, I had to remember that this event was temporary, local and changeable. Martin Seligman, the father of positive psychology, discovered that people who don't give up and interpret setbacks as temporary, local, and changeable, are more immune to helplessness, depression and anxiety than those who see catastrophe everywhere.

The idea is that the specific moment or experience is 'temporary'. It is going away soon; it will pass and it will not last forever. The temporary sense of the experience or event might be just a fleeting moment, when you recognise that the sun is out, the pain (whether that be mental, emotional or physical) has changed or reduced. The exact experience you are in is not forever.

Identifying the experience as 'local' brings in the context around the situation. The specific experience does not need to be all-encompassing. Seeing the bigger picture of life by observing the environment, the people, the situations, the conversations, and the varying roles one plays, is one way to notice the many different contexts or parts of life. Identifying one tough experience as local, creates a sense of control and ease in life.

The third step in this concept is interpreting the situation as 'changeable'. It means things can change, move, vary, or transform. The one thing we have control over is our thoughts. We can change the way we think about a situation even if we cannot change the actual event. The best part of identifying the experience as changeable is that we can take back our power (no matter how big or small). It means we are not stuck, stagnant and have no options available.

For me, taking time to slow down, reduce the stimulation (mentally and physically) and check-in with myself, was important for my recovery after a year of being worn down mentally, physically and emotionally. This included being in a toxic work environment, having plummeting iron levels, two bouts of surgery, and the daily interactions, constant appointments and treatment.

The daily exposure to constant stimulation was extreme. This included hospital visits with others who were on their own out-of-control life-threatening journeys; excessive amounts of adrenaline and cortisol rushing through my body; appointments and interactions with Oncologists, Radiotherapists and other medical staff; and lying under a machine the size of a small house that was emanating whirring and buzzing sounds. This was on top of my usual daily tasks of just living.

During periods when my physical body was reacting negatively to the radiation treatment I went into lockdown to preserve my energy. As the course of radiation treatment continued, I did not receive a great deal of goodness from any food as it was going straight through me. During the treatment I experienced diarrhea and developed intolerances to many food groups, as predicted by the medical staff.

As the impact of the treatment accumulated, the side effects increased. I became more aware of where and when I was going out. Would it include mealtimes (which were very challenging in terms of food types and preferences), was there a decent bathroom available if I needed it, and would I be with someone who was understanding enough to tolerate my needs? These changes in habits and the impact of the side effects had me feeling very dependent on people when I was out and about.

Physically I wasn't working out or exercising as much as I usually would, and this took its toll on me mentally and physically. I was used to working out at least three times per week, if not more, and being very active in between these times. However, due to the radiotherapy and its side effects, as well as recovering from surgery, I was having to lockdown physically as well. I had down time during the day when I would often have a sleep, take time to lie down and listen to music, read or just 'be'. This initial lockdown time during treatment was the three months following surgery, so it was a mixture of recovery and going through radiotherapy at the same time.

Recharging my battery was something I always did physically, so this was a very challenging time. I had to deal with the fact of not being able to recharge in my usual way, yet I had to find a way to be able to recharge that would get me through the demanding situation.

My natural 'go to' when I need a pick me up or to calm down is initially something physical and then to learn something new. Working out new ways to respond to this demanding situation was causing a great deal of conflicting thoughts for me such as, "If I can't work out or do something physical then I'm doomed", "Maybe if I did a little bit of physical training then I'd be ok, but if I do any physical work I'll ruin the good recovery I'm making".

Chapter 10

Controlling the Controllables

T he new normal was cemented into my life every day of my recovery, and it was my choice whether to accept and make sense of this, or to resist and *fight* it. Many people kept telling me to fight cancer, to battle on. To me it makes no sense to *fight*. If I fight anything, then I am adding to the negativity of the situation. I am actually fighting MYSELF!

If I engage my energy in fighting what is happening to me, I sap any energy that I could use to heal my body and close down possibilities to enjoy the moments of happiness in life. Why would I fight myself and the situation I am in? There are many areas of my life affected by this past experience. Some will be with me forever, and some hopefully will fade with time. I am growing in physical strength and energy every month.

One strategy I used during this journey was *three good things and why*. This evidence-based tactic was developed by Martin Seligman and his team (2005). It is writing down three good things that you have experienced in the last 24 hours and identify *why* they happened.

This could be as small as enjoying a delicious tasting coffee. An action that I developed into a ceremonial moment. It was a *good thing* because I allowed myself to slow down and engage my senses as I felt, smelt and tasted each mouthful purposefully. The warmth of the cup, the aroma of the beverage, and finally, the scintillating taste of coffee (double shot skinny piccolo please).

A bigger example is receiving the donations on GoFundMe® with the most amazing messages of support. The *why*? Regardless of the monetary value, one very personal message stands out with a small donation that was huge for the giver, and was written with heartfelt meaning, love and vulnerability. A blessing to receive.

The reason why the strategy of three good things is so powerful is that it increases positive emotions and decreases negative emotions. It also shifts our focus from things that go wrong, or having lack or scarcity, to things that we can appreciate and be grateful for. Writing down the causes of *the three good things* allows us to reflect in detail about the quality of the experience, increases self-awareness, and raises our overall satisfaction with life.

This daily strategy is incredibly powerful when we reflect on the positive events in our day with gratitude and savour each moment. This intentional savouring allows us to slow down, be fully present, and have a strong sense of meaning beyond ourselves.

When faced with an uncontrollable moment, our response is the only thing we can control. To be at our best in these moments is tough and we need to be honest with ourselves and others, choose optimistic language, and elicit strong positive connections with people in our environment.

There will be many unknowns in our lives that elicit fear, emotions, and force us to shape a response. The challenge is to draw on those strengths, skills and abilities that we have learned from every moment in our past. This will enable us to launch forth with limitless possibilities into the unknown and learn to flourish!

When you come to the end of your rope, tie a knot in it and hang on!
– Franklin D Roosevelt –

Martin Seligman, as Director of the Penn Master of Applied Positive Psychology program (MAPP), also identified that flourishing is more than just happiness or wellbeing. Flourishing is the key to improving the quality of life for people around the world. It encompasses a wide range of positive psychology paradigms and offers a more holistic perspective on what it means to feel well and happy.

Flourishing includes all experiences, regardless of the interpretation we give them. It incorporates positive and negative emotions and all of life events. Barbara Fredrickson, Professor of Psychology and the *broaden and build* theorist, espouses that the secret to flourishing in life is to have a ratio of at least 3:1 (2013); three positive emotions for every one negative emotion.

Some recent literature in this area suggests the ratio is even higher at 5:1. This means if you receive negative feedback for something you have done or failed to do, you need to bring to mind three positive things you have, are, or do to counteract the impact of the negative. This embeds the positive effects, deepens the meaning, and allows you to stay in the moment longer.

My example is: The test results stated I had cancer (a negative); the three positives - a great conversation with the surgeon, a delicious coffee, some wonderful flowers blooming in the garden on the way to the hospital. When I was able to instigate the three to one method, I built my resilience and moved towards flourishing in that moment.

The ability to flourish in life is when individuals experience high levels of PERMA in daily life, defined as *Positive Emotion, Engagement, Relationships, Meaning* and *Accomplishment* (Seligman, 2012). We need to increase our positive emotions (P), engage with the world and our activities (E), have deep and meaningful relationships (R), find meaning and purpose in our lives (M), and accomplish our goals (A).

This approach to life was developed from research carried out by Martin Seligman describing five core elements that assist people to reach a life of fulfilment, happiness and meaning (Seligman, 2012). A flourishing person has all five elements of PERMA present in their life and is aiming to maximise each element where possible. Enabling each of these elements in everyday life facilitates happiness, wellbeing and resilience.

This can all happen when we cultivate our abilities and apply our innate strengths to everything we do. I trained myself to apply the theory of PERMA to gain more optimism and engage positive strategies during this adverse event.

The first element of PERMA is **Positive Emotion** – this is more than just happiness or 'being positive'. Positive emotions include things like love, joy, amusement, compassion, gratitude and pride. An individual's ability to experience positive emotions is a combination of genetic makeup, identifying things with gratitude, and focusing on the positive aspects of various experiences. When we stop and allow ourselves to contemplate the moment (look back with gladness and forward with hope and excitement), we are savouring an experience.

We notice the positives in a situation or imagine the future with an optimistic approach, therefore strengthening the element of positive emotion. Optimism is the belief that you will generally experience positive outcomes in life. People with higher levels of optimism are more resilient to stressful life events. A systematic review with meta-analysis (to determine the significant findings that worked) into optimism and physical health reported that people who have an optimistic approach to life, live longer, have less sickness, are physically healthier and have improved post-operative outcomes (Rasmussen, Scheier & Greenhouse, 2009).

Research has also identified that a purposeful focus on positive emotions can undo the effects of negative emotions, help prevent illness, and speed up recovery from ill health (Seligman, 2011). Taking time each day to identify things that you are grateful for will help to build positive emotions and increase an optimistic approach. Additional strategies can include spending quality time with people you care about and enjoy being with, having times of laughter, doing activities that you enjoy, listening to uplifting music, or engaging in physical exercise.

Positive emotions can be tested in times of adversity. If habits and routines change because of an event, then it is difficult to maintain our usual positive emotions, gratitude, or optimism. When routines and habits are undergoing changes, incorporating the elements of PERMA eases the effects of negative emotions, reduces stress, reduces recovery time and promotes resilience.

Visiting the hospital five out of seven days a week for six weeks isn't a usual routine for most of the population, unless you happen to work there. Finding optimism in an undesirable activity or task like this can be a constructive way to help reduce the negative emotional investment. Linking positive thoughts, feelings and experiences to an adjustment in routine is beneficial to maintaining a sense of control and self-efficacy.

I constantly reminded myself that the times I spent at the hospital were when I could be a joy germ and spread happiness to others. It was a time when I could dedicate myself to mindfulness whilst on the radiotherapy bed, and a time to receive the devoted skills, abilities and compassion of the experts, which instilled hope and improved health.

During a time of adversity, as challenging as it may seem, the best thing to do is accept the situation *as-is* (optimism), have faith in ourselves and the team around us, and believe there will be an end point (hope). Being real in the moment increases the ability to problem solve, raises levels of happiness, decreases levels of stress, and creates a less traumatic way forward. Whereas seeing a situation as too hard, too big or too challenging, reduces our ability to problem-solve and leads to repeating the same negative patterns.

As humans we often need to consciously remind ourselves to take a moment and focus on the positive rather than the negative aspects in life. This can be a challenge as the human brain is wired to connect and focus on the negative. Research experiments have shown that the brain typically reacts more strongly to *perceived* negative stimuli. The way we perceive and make sense of the world is through our beliefs, intelligence, experiences and the development of our mental processes.

However, the good news is that studies have reported we can rewire our brains over time to perceive events, experiences and situations as positive (Ito, Larsen, Smith, & Cacioppo, 1998). Even if we have a negative approach, there are ways we can change this perception and be more positive in life.

To assist in increasing the positive emotions during times of change or adversity, take a few minutes each day to consciously redirect your thoughts towards three good experiences in the past 24 hours. These experiences may have been positive, happy, valuable, or pleasant. This can be small or large; a delicious coffee, a beautiful sunset through to a career promotion, or getting engaged. Either in thought, spoken, or in writing, this shifts the focus from negative to positive.

In addition, it is beneficial to reflect on *why* the experience was good. This takes the activity a step further by embedding the positive emotion on a deeper level. You get to decide the reasons for each event being a good one, i.e. not judged by anyone else. It is a totally personal experience and interpretation. Examples may incorporate, "I connected with our conversation so much more because I didn't use my phone", "I was looking forward to my coffee at my favourite café". By re-focusing on a moment in the day that is good we will increase positive emotions.

The second element of PERMA is **Engagement**. This is described as *being one* with the activity. Time tends to stop and we become less self-conscious. We lose track of time when we are fully engaged in things we enjoy doing, that are at the right level of demand for our abilities. This means we are living in the present moment and entirely focused on the task at hand. This is also known as *flow*, being *in the zone* or being in an *ideal performance state*.

The leading researcher in this field of engagement in flow is Mihaly Csikszentmihalyi (2011). He states:

> "The best moments in our lives are not the passive, receptive,
> relaxing times… The best moments usually occur if a person's
> body or mind is stretched to its limits in a voluntary effort to
> accomplish something difficult and worthwhile." (p.3)

We experience flow when our greatest innate strengths are truly and deeply engaged during a challenging task. These strengths are defined as natural, and they are authentic resources that represent what is good in each of us (Langley & Francis, 2015). Examples include creativity, learning, persistence, kindness, and humility (Seligman, 2011).

Studies have identified that when individuals incorporate their innate strengths into their daily activities, or are in a state of flow, they are happier, more productive, significantly less stressed and experience higher levels of mental, physical and emotional wellbeing (Csikszentmihalyi, 2011).

When we engage in tasks that we love doing so that we lose track of time and have very little self-conscious awareness, we are building our engagement and increasing the moments of flow. This can also be done through practising mindfulness or meditation and doing activities like yoga or tai chi. The reason for this is that we calm down the chatter in the mind, and re-focus our internal ideas, thoughts, attitudes and feelings.

When practising these activities we are training ourselves to become very aware of every thought and body process. This ripples into other areas of our lives so that we can experience flow more often and more deeply. We can then become very aware of what we are doing at any point in time. We are totally present and absorbed in that specific moment. Appreciating and savouring the *now* enables us to become present. By consciously taking the time to focus on and be engaged with the present moment we can build the level of engagement and flow that we experience.

The third element of PERMA is ***Relationships***. Social connections are one of the most important aspects of human life. They have a significant impact on wellbeing. It's how humans are constructed. Cultivating positive relationships with people supports us to function within a community and sets up the opportunity to give joy, love and happiness to others. This is a relationship of reciprocity. When surrounded by supportive people we are more likely to become content and joyful.

There are different levels of positive connection – strong or superficial. Having strong connections with individuals provides a support network when going through tough times. Research has identified that strong support networks positively assist an individual's recovery and improve health outcomes (Gosnell & Gable, 2017). When we are supported by strong social connections, our physical, mental, and emotional health is enhanced so we experience higher levels of health and wellbeing. To enhance our relationships and therefore boost our health and happiness, it is vital that we are open to both giving and receiving.

The way I chose to give to others post-diagnosis was acknowledging and talking with every person from the carpark to the treatment area. This included random visitors, other patients, cleaning staff, administration staff, security staff and support people. I always wanted to take this connection beyond the superficial, and most often connected on a deeper level.

Some interactions quickly took on a very deep connection, like the 82-year-old man discussing his cancer diagnosis, recent loss of his wife to cancer, and his respect for women and their pelvic floors. We were complete strangers, talking about *our bits* and offering each other support in this difficult time.

I took it on myself to look out for the people who were super anxious and obvious newbies. I could sense their fear and worked to assist with allaying this with them through building connection. I slowly felt more in tune with how the whole game worked. There are no real rules of what to say or do when going through a traumatic event. Saying hello to strangers is a way to increase our connections with others and strengthen community. Even though this can be scary, when feeling fearful, scared or stressed, a positive interaction can have an immediate affirming physical, mental and emotional impact on both the giver and the recipient.

I was so blessed to receive during this time through my strong relationships and connections. From my wife I received everything. Devotion and every piece of emotional, physical and mental support, even though she was struggling within this time too. She gave me everything, every ounce of her energy, her love and every part of her.

I felt so bad because during these times I was helpless, and could not reciprocate because I was physically and emotionally unable. But I guess this is what strong connections are about – giving and receiving in different ways to the capacity and ability of the person at the time.

I received love and joy from others as well, to bolster me up when it was tough. The support varied from timely words such as "Go you", "Keep going", "Don't give up", to deep genuine concern with action. Some of the deeper gifts included money to support the bills, treats to celebrate poignant milestones, doing things for me that were true to who I was and what I needed, deep and meaningful messages that were incredibly personal and displayed how much they knew me, and gifts that were given at great personal cost. Being open to receiving these gifts supported my wellbeing and contributed to my ability to bounce forward during this difficult time.

I hadn't yet shared this journey with my sister, nephews and niece. We hadn't really had a strong connection in recent years and this was tricky, but I knew I needed to tell them that I had been diagnosed with cancer. I really struggled with this. Dad had died from cancer and Mum was a breast cancer survivor but died soon after from other causes.

I didn't want them to worry, get upset or think that I was going to die - even though I didn't really know what the definite prognosis was. I knew sharing the information was good for me. It would shift me from my struggle to admitting what was happening, and allow me the opportunity to grow my support team. I did not know how they would respond. How they chose to respond was out of my control and it was up to them to react in their own way.

It had become my role in the family to be tough, always in control, healthy and the one who sorted things out. This was a lot of pressure. I thought I was protecting them by not speaking up, and didn't want to deal with any strange responses. Being real and showing my vulnerability was something that scared me at various times during this journey, and this was one of them. There were various responses to my disclosure.

They were what they were. We are still a family and are working to build stronger connections.

As I shared my story, expressed my real feelings, and admitted the hugeness of this traumatic event, my relationships with those in my *team* grew stronger. My emotional and physical health also strengthened. I discovered that vulnerability was my new weapon to finding good health.

Sometimes people didn't know what to say or do, so they did nothing. This was hurtful at the time for me in the middle of the trauma, and has changed some of these relationships. Some have fallen away, and others are much more prominent and meaningful in my everyday life. I have learned throughout this journey that relationships have to be a deep and meaningful two-way connection. Knowing that relationships have such a huge impact on health and happiness (physically and emotionally) I invest in the relationships that are going to work positively for both parties.

We all have limited time and energy on this planet and to thrive as an individual we need to build strong connections and relationships that give and receive in order to flourish within a community of love and support.

The fourth element of PERMA is ***Meaning***. To gain a sense of meaning we need to feel that what we do is valuable and worthwhile. Having a purpose, belonging to or serving something higher than ourselves is how meaning links to our health and happiness. Finding our meaning in life may be in the work we do beyond paid employment, it may be the contribution we make in our daily roles, a political involvement, a voluntary position, a spiritual belief, or a cause we are passionate about.

Research in this area has identified that those who have a strong sense of meaning show higher levels of happiness and are also more likely to respond to adversity with greater resilience (Seligman, 2011). This sets us up to discover who we really are, what we are about, and hooks into a deeper understanding of self. When we find a greater sense of meaning beyond self, we experience a deeper sense of worth known as post-traumatic growth (Tedeschi & Calhoun, 2016).

This is when survivors of traumatic events can not only heal from their trauma, but grow into a stronger, more driven and more resilient person.

Identifying what is important to us comes through experiencing trauma. It is often in these times of adversity that we start to determine our reason to exist in life. People who have a strong reason to live have greater satisfaction and fewer health problems (Diener & Chan 2011). When people feel in alignment with their purpose and a higher sense of meaning, they will have more interest in the activity, contribute more, and have increased levels of function and wellbeing.

To enhance our meaning in life it is important to spend time in, contribute to, engage in and connect with activities, people and reasons that are authentic to us. Find your purpose, find the things that make you smile, and commit to your involvement in these daily. When adversity or challenges strike it is important for your mental, physical and emotional health to keep participating and contributing to this meaning beyond self.

I wanted to find meaning within my set routines of turning up to the hospital every day for treatment. I decided to make these times an opportunity to contribute to others beyond myself. I was unsure what else I could do, how much energy I had for others, or what else I could physically accomplish. I needed to link into something I was good at doing in order to contribute.

For me this was being a joy germ and connecting with people. This was about being and doing something I was good at, something that came naturally so that I could contribute within my restricted limits of energy. Thinking and contributing to others in this way stopped me from getting caught up in my own response to the trauma. It got me out of my own thoughts and distracted me from these negative emotions.

I also knew that this was a scientific way to change the chemicals in my mind and body and therefore help with my own healing and wellbeing. When we are open, self-aware and receptive to contributing to others within our abilities, we are highly likely to be able to adapt, learn and grow during adversity and explore our sense of meaning in new and exciting ways.

The fifth and final element of PERMA is ***Accomplishment***. This is also known as achievement or mastery. Having a sense of accomplishment means that we have worked towards and reached a target or goal. Pursuing goals that match our personal values and interests makes it easier to achieve them.

Achieving goals has been shown to enhance wellbeing and increase optimism (Seligman, 2011; Duckworth, 2016). Accomplishment is a contributing factor to our wellbeing in the sense that we can reflect back and say *I did it*. This recognition of achievement releases endorphins (e.g. serotonin, dopamine, oxytocin) which increases muscle strength, cognitive acuity, and can lead us to a state of flow and self-worth. These responses can be addictive in that you want to continue to push yourself to achieve more and more.

Every time I went to treatment, I felt so good about the responses I received so I wanted to give more. They chatted, shared and connected with me on deeper levels. I felt like I was doing good. I was contributing something to others which counteracted the negative experiences without me realising it, and gave me a sense of normality. This balanced the feelings of trauma and uncertainty in these moments.

Small tastes of success are required to achieve goals and strengthen one's ability to persevere. Set yourself up to achieve not fail, and be aware of self-sabotage. Learn, grow and develop in the pursuit of achievement and mastery. Always look for ways to celebrate those achievements no matter how small they are. Express your achievement with others and savour the accomplishments. This will increase your interest and validate the alignment of the goals with your values. Set yourself up for success.

I made the choice to take control by implementing the elements of PERMA into my life as I began to discover, create and build my new normal. This adverse event had thrust me into a situation where I could decide to instigate a *new* approach and bounce forward, or allow life to pass me by while I remained stuck in the trauma of negative emotion.

A mix of PERMA and gratitude (being thankful for what you have, right here, right now) are the important things in life to keep you healthy and happy. This is the tipping point which will help determine whether you languish in life or flourish. When you choose to flourish you live a life full of possibilities and become more resilient in the tough times.

I chose to implement PERMA and take the optimistic approach to bounce forward with resilience. The challenge for YOU is will you choose the same regardless of what the adversity is today?

"To flourish is to find fulfillment in our lives, accomplishing meaning and worthwhile tasks, and connecting to others at a deeper level"
– Martin Seligman

Chapter 11

Reclaiming Power

In the beginning of my journey I was understandably uncertain of how I needed to respond to the situation I was in, so I sought to find answers. I had been aware of Dr Carol Dweck, a Professor at Stanford University, and her studies into human motivation. She explores why people succeed or don't, and how they cultivate success (2017). She discovered that what we can identify as being 'within our control', is the key to resilience and motivation to achieve.

Her theory is based on the notion that an individual's mindset (a person's self-conceptions that guide behaviour) either *prevents* them from fulfilling their potential or *propels* them to learn, grow and develop. This is stated as either a fixed mindset or a growth mindset (Dweck, 2017). Neuroscience has shown that we can shift from a fixed mindset towards a growth mindset. If you identify that you have a fixed mindset approach in a specific area of your life, this can be transformed to become a growth mindset through effort and action.

A **fixed mindset** is the understanding that intelligence and qualities cannot be developed, they are fixed traits. They are carved in stone. The hand you have been dealt is unchangeable and there is no way of growing or developing. An individual with this mindset invests in negative thoughts, rejects new ideas, gives up in the face of adversity, is inflexible, avoids challenges, ignores useful feedback, feels threatened by the success of others, and chases mediocrity.

Engaging in life with a fixed mindset harnesses thoughts and actions of constantly wanting to prove oneself correct over and over again, instead of learning from mistakes. This stems from the belief that we have been dealt a terrible hand of luck, scarcity, illness or life drama. This negatively impacts on all areas of life. As a result, the individual may plateau in life at an early age and achieve less than their full potential. All this confirms a deterministic view of the world, where the external determines what and how we achieve.

A fixed mindset person is highly sensitive to being wrong or making a mistake, and avoids this at all costs. Failure will enhance our self-doubt and destroy confidence. As a result, we will feel anxious and fragile when receiving setbacks and criticisms. When we have a low level of confidence, believe we are powerless and cannot change the situation, then our resilience is undermined. With a low level of resilience, we are open to more negative situations, which lessens the likelihood of putting in more effort to change any situation.

A **growth mindset** is the understanding that one's abilities and intelligence to learning, effort and practice can be developed (Dweck, 2017). This mindset believes that it is not simply about the hand we have been dealt in life but the ability to change this. The situation we are in is only the starting point. From this point we can grow, develop, and create a better way of life.

This leads to the desire to learn and therefore a tendency to do this; as well as embrace challenges, persist in the face of setbacks, see effort as the path to mastery, learn from criticism, and find lessons and inspiration in the success of others. As a result, we will reach higher levels of achievement, sustain a greater sense of power, and strengthen our self-identity. This is the mindset that allows people to thrive (develop, grow, prosper, flourish) during the most challenging times.

Dr Dweck and her colleagues at Stanford tested the correlation between mindset and self-identity with patients who had breast cancer (n=20) in a longitudinal study (Horst, Fero, Haimovitz & Dweck 2012). They reported that those with a fixed mindset had low levels of self-identity, high emotional distress, and a perception that cancer was taking over their life. Those with a growth mindset had high levels of self-identity resulting in less distress and an ability to pursue life purposefully. This also translated into higher resilience and persistence in the face of a setback.

Growth mindset is associated with the drive for stretching ourselves and persevering, particularly when things are not going well (resilience). When we engage in resilient behaviour and take ownership of the situation (regain power) then we are likely to thrive in life.

Thriving with a growth mindset includes being courageous enough to explore possible solutions and not give up. Dweck discusses that there are two defined paradigms we engage in when a situation is 'too hard' to solve right now:
1) Are you not smart enough to solve it? Or
2) Have you just not solved it 'yet'?

If we don't have the skills to solve a situation then we need to address this and find some help. The use of the term 'yet' opens up the idea that future changes are possible and assists with exploring solutions. We have not given up but are finding a way through adversity. People with a growth mindset flourish in life, open up to their fears, change and adapt to situations, embrace challenges, and see disappointments or disasters as an opportunity to evolve.

From the day of 'the phone call', I decided that I would adapt mentally, physically and emotionally to whatever was about to happen. I would take control of what I was able to control (internal locus of control), and the medical team could take charge of and control the medical treatment in order to destroy the cancer cells (external locus of control).

The *locus of control* principle considers the tendency of individuals to believe that control resides internally within them, or externally with others or the situation. In 1954, psychologist Julian Rotter coined the term 'locus of control' to refer to people's beliefs about what causes good or bad things to happen in their lives (Rotter, 1954). This is similar to theoretical approaches which are set on a fluid continuum (i.e. growth and fixed mindset) where people are not inflexible on one or the other extremes. We have an overall tendency for a preference to one end of the continuum, however this can change depending on life circumstances, age, health, demands, unfamiliar or constant factors.

A person with a high *internal* locus of control believes in their ability to control themselves and influence the world around them (Rotter, 1966). They see the future as being in their own hands, and their choices lead directly to success or failure. They take responsibility for mistakes, see them as learning opportunities and have the ability to separate situations to deal with each one individually.

People with a high *external* locus of control believe they have no influence over events, situations or people. They are powerless to make anything change for themselves. These individuals believe that luck, chance or fate is the reason for most outcomes. If they receive anything 'good', there is no acknowledgement that they influenced, created or worked to gain this - it was just fate or luck. If 'bad' things happen they perceive this as bad luck, the 'story of my life', and have an inability to change this. A common adage is 'why me, what have I done to deserve this'? These people tend to be fatalistic, pre-determined, and view things as happening TO them.

This was not going to be me. I reclaimed that I was in charge of controlling my internal thoughts and reactions to be able to take back my power over this uncontrollable situation. Even though I had made this decision, there were times during my recovery I felt like there were many things that were happening to me.

An example of this is how I moved from internal to external at different times throughout my journey of recovery. I completed Rotter's locus of control questionnaire (1966) in March 2016 during my year of declining health and scored a very strong tendency towards *internal* locus of control. This is indicative of previous scores I have had throughout my life.

However, throughout this journey there were times of oscillation from internal to external in the depths of feeling powerless. I identified that there were so many things beyond my control, more external input on what I could or could not do than ever before, and my internal locus of control was wavering. I recognised that it was time to reignite my skills and abilities to get this back to the high level that it had always been. I needed to take my power back, take action and once again, control the controllables.

My plan was to start small and focus on one thing at a time. This meant looking at my current roles and responsibilities and identifying what capabilities (mental, physical and emotional) I still possessed to begin taking my power back. I selected one action that I could achieve. This was to engage and connect with the people I met at the treatment centre. I didn't need to exert physical energy but I could alter the direction of my emotions and contribute to others.

My second small action was to do something physical. I slowly began to be able to prepare dinner for us both. This gave me a sense of contributing to our home life and taking back a small part of my role and its responsibilities.

Setting up win-win-win situations (for me, others, and a positive outcome) was judicious. Making contributions to people, preparing dinner, listening to others, and making deeper connections was paramount. This embodied empowering myself to be authentic and inspiring others to follow their own authenticity.

Taking small steps every day to increase my resilience was extremely important. The actions I took every single day were to follow my routine so that mentally and physically my body was in the best state for treatment.

I would drink the required amount of water so the radiotherapy treatment could hit its target. I would dress tidily to go to the hospital to maintain my self-respect and feel good about the way I looked. I arrived early for each treatment to be respectful of the staff's time, and allowed for any traffic delays. I would always look the staff in the eye and greet them warmly. I would engage in my three to one ritual (refer chapter 10) with other patients in the waiting areas. I folded my clothes neatly as I put them into the basket and got changed into my crease-free gown with pride. I had that gown for 30 treatments and it looked great the entire time. After each treatment had finished, I would take satisfaction in folding up my gown and knowing that was treatment done for the day. My gown represented part of who I was, and it was another small part of something I could control every single day of my treatment. It was my uniform for this treatment game and I needed to 'look good and play well'.

I needed to have a plan in place to manage the 'private number' phone calls. My strategy was to find out exactly why they had rung, get the best option for myself for the appointment, and feel like I had been recognised as ME on the phone call. If it took using the person's name several times, being light-hearted about the situation, sharing something positive, or talking with the person in a way that showed the realness of the situation, then that's what I did. This didn't stop the instant fear arising from the 'private number' call, but it enabled me to find a way through the fear.

There was a chunk of me that needed to let go of doubts and fears, otherwise I would not play well. I needed to let go of the desire to control everything with the realisation that I didn't know how long I would be on this Earth and needed to enjoy what life I had left. It's a strange feeling when you are forced to comprehend your mortality - scary and beyond your control.

I needed to let go of the fears, which was very hard to do. I knew I could not control the future so needed to stop thinking this was somehow possible, and be vulnerable enough to be human and embrace my impermanence. There was no room for excuses, delay tactics or waiting. I had to act now. Letting go of all these reactions, which I initially thought I needed to keep, and allow a specialist in their field who had my best interests at heart to step into my life and call the shots, was imperative. Strange… yes, weird… yes, difficult… extremely. It was totally opposite to what I usually think and do, but was now a requirement for me to regain my power in life.

During this transition time, I was willing to make a 'trade-off'. A trade-off is the exchange of one thing at the expense of another, and is a way of making sense of loss and pain with the benefit of making choices. For example, I knew the probable outcomes of consuming certain foods. They reacted with my compromised digestive system and caused uncomfortable side effects.

Four specific foods (cheese, olives, cold meats and pickled vegetables) were on this list, however at times I was willing to accept the consequences of ingesting these in return for the pleasurable event of connecting with others. I chose an upsetting physiological response in order to have a moment of normality with my wife and family. There was no doubt about the negative consequences, and I was fully aware of them when making the decision.

The flavours, the aromas and the textures of those foods were amazing. I had been eating clean, bland foods for several weeks and just wanted to experience the connection of food and senses. That moment was like being free of dis-ease; it was a moment of contentedness. The cancer diagnosis did not own me, it was part of me and I was still me. This was a moment to exert my *emotional flexibility*. I knew I would recover within two to three days after allowing myself this trade-off and it was worth it. I trusted myself to make these decisions.

Trust became a major factor in this new chapter of life. Trust is both a logical thought and an emotional act. It involves calculating the risk of vulnerability where we are confident enough to expose ourselves to others without fear of reprisal or hurt. Without trust we are not able to thrive and flourish, maintain deep and meaningful connections, or contribute to others. Trust is linked with levels of subjective wellbeing, and when one decreases so does the other (Tay & Diener, 2011). Trusting ourselves, and trusting others who may hold our life in their hands is essential.

Trust can often be challenging. For me people have to earn my trust; it is not automatic. For others, they trust until the person gives them a reason not to. It is important to know our stance on 'trust' and this will be something to carry forward through times of adversity. We tend to trust people who share common beliefs and values.

Trust is developed over time, enabling us to take risks, express feelings, share ideas and act in a more confident way because we know someone 'has our back'. When we trust, our stress levels go down and levels of good health and happiness rise. Having faith and trust in someone on our team allows us to achieve more, recover more quickly, be at our best, and invest time in the activities we need or want.

I discovered this involved trusting my intuition, which is the little voice inside us that says "Watch out, something is not right", or "Yes this is a good person to trust". I was not used to trusting my intuition in an overt way and often ignored this in the past. When we acknowledge and follow our intuition, we are often more confident to step forward and feel safe to explore the options.

The feeling of safety was important to me throughout the journey, and still is when I am back at the hospital for check-ups, visits or interactions regarding this experience. Sometimes I have to tell myself, "They are the experts, they know what they are doing" and allow myself to step back and feel safe in their hands (trust). I follow my intuition and take control of the controllables at each appointment, like how I present myself, how I interact, and the information I request.

I developed a mutual trust between myself and my team. They had faith and trust in me that I would follow their instructions, and I had faith in them to do what was best for my health with positive outcomes. When we are being our best in any situation by showing our vulnerabilities, being our authentic self, allowing people to speak into our lives and trusting our intuition, we will get the most out of life.

There may be countless moments when this stretches us and tests our resolve in every fibre of our bodies. It is our choice whether we allow 'them' to take over and control us, which leads to a feeling of disempowerment, or to regain control and initiate positive actions. This is the time to instigate our growth mindset, take back our power, trust ourselves and others, and build our resilience.

There is always a lesson to be learned in any situation if we are open to it. Apart from seeming like a pile of clichés, I have learnt so much about myself, my strengths, my tenacity and determination, and am now in a totally different place four years after that day. I have seen, heard and experienced situations that have enabled me to choose a fresh perspective on life. Those experiences and learnings wouldn't have happened if I had stayed powerless. This entire experience has been a gift, one that has given me a strength of character I did not have before, and is with me forever.

It really is in the toughest times that we grow the most.

Your limitless possibilities...

1) Listen to your mind and body
   - Recognise and feel the change in body sensations
   - Hear/feel/see the messages from your body and respond positively
2) Control the controllables
   - Recognise the thoughts in your head
   - Take charge of your thoughts, feelings and actions
3) Write down three good things and why they occurred, each day
   - Gratitude changes perception, so keep a record of three things each day (no matter how small or big these may seem)
   - Every little win counts!
4) Identify if you have more of a Fixed or Growth mindset
   - Engage your growth mindset
   - Embrace challenges as opportunities
   - Learn something new each day
5) Shift into your Internal locus of control
   - Take responsibility for mistakes and achievements
6) Reframe your doubts and fears
   - Identify what these are, reframe them

7) Trust yourself and others
- Trust your intuition
- Create a solid support team

8) Take back your Power!

Section Four

PURPOSEFUL INTENTION

* * *

Affirmation: "I am what I think and believe"

Chapter 12

Gameplan Discovery

I had a choice – I could either feel sorry for myself and disengage from people and activities, or I could keep going every single day. At least the treatment only targeted my abdominal and pelvic regions, it was not about the whole of my body. The disruption to my life and the things I wanted to do was not forever. If I kept going I knew there would eventually be an end point and everything would be fine. Deep within there was certainty that I would get through this. Somehow and in some way the treatment, the process and the outcomes would change.

People may define this as creating the new normal, but to me, it was just what I had to do. For now, the treatment and new life routines would become my new normal; a place where I could adapt to the new daily demands. If I didn't adapt and find new strategies, I was going to do more harm to my life than good.

My treatment schedule meant an upheaval of our plans for Christmas, and we also had to cancel a booked holiday. The intensity of the situation was brought home to us when I had to attend a daily treatment on

Christmas Eve. While other people were meeting up with friends and family, eating out, going on holiday, shopping and planning festivities, we went to the hospital, sat in a dark, dingy hole and waited to be called in for treatment. Instead of being outdoors enjoying new adventures, for the next two weeks we were forced to turn up and face the realities of the diagnosis. I had no control over the treatment timetable. We were given their designated times, and there was no consideration for holidays or occasions.

This timetable continued over the holiday period and even affected New Year festivities. Instead of doing what we had planned, due to fatigue I was unable to stay out late, be around too much noise, or socialise for long periods. We attended the children's fireworks at 9 p.m. so I could be with Elizabeth to enjoy seeing in some aspect of the New Year.

Christmas and New Year of 2016/2017 will be forever marked by preparation routines, attending treatment, and experiencing fatigue as it started to set in. One bright moment was building a 3D jigsaw model of the Eiffel Tower, which even had a changing lights phase. This was a great achievement for us both, although Elizabeth did the fiddly stuff as my hands were a bit big. Even now when I look at the 3D Tower sitting proudly in our lounge, I smile and embrace that joyous moment of achievement.

During this time of adversity I was able to be present, and have moments of joy and accomplishment. Even though I wasn't in control of most of the process, it was good to be reminded that there were some things within it that I could control.

Physical activity majorly decreased due to fatigue. Having always been active it was tough for me to adjust to not doing what I wanted to do. I consistently felt like I was dragging myself through mud, which made me grumpy, then knew this would impact Elizabeth. I wanted to stop and to keep going at the same time, but just couldn't. It became a vicious cycle of desire, expectation, compromise and failure. I became even more highly tuned into my body, mentally, physically and emotionally, and had to gauge the length of time, degree of stimulation and exertion that every task required in every single moment.

There were also certain expectations from others about what I 'should' be able to do or not do, and what I was actually capable of doing during this time. Some overestimated my abilities while others grossly underestimated them. This totally annoyed me as I was unable to carry on 'as usual' and they didn't understand the impact and side effects of the treatment for me.

Sometimes the nurses predicted the worse-case scenario and were surprised when this didn't happen. While others expected me to be a total cot case on my deathbed, when I wasn't they thought I was faking it. Why didn't they just let me be and talk about what I needed? Everyone has different abilities, capacities and thresholds during adverse situations, and if this isn't happening to you directly, then be open enough to ask and find out what is happening for the person.

During this time my way of maintaining control and allowing the 'new normal' to be shaped, was to go into my 'sporting mode'. This involved narrowing my focus in order to block out superfluous things, and turning on all my senses so I could react quickly to whatever was required. I had a resounding belief in myself that I could do this and would come out on top, which is how I always think, talk and behave in order to perform at my best. Being an optimist, I identified the positives that were already in my life and the benefits I was gaining from this experience.

To be at my best I had to engage my 'pre-performance routine'. When I woke up I smiled with all my being, sat up and drank a glass of water, went to the bathroom, and then drank the required fluids for treatment. I knew if I drank the right amount of water, my bladder would be in the right place to minimise damage. Next, I would shower with the purposeful intent of being clean and refreshed. I would also apply my favourite deodorant and perfume so I would smell and feel good. Then I would do my makeup and dress up slightly, believing that if I looked good I wasn't a victim of the situation. If I looked good, felt good and smelled good, then I would perform well and be at my best.

Felicia Huppert, the Founder and Director of the Wellbeing Institute at Cambridge University, puts it simply by stating that when we engage in enhancing our wellbeing, which includes boosting our resilience, we will 'feel good and function well'. For me it gave me a sense of control over the controllables, so I could focus on the immediate situation and reduce worry or anxiety. This had worked for me so many times in the past with sport so I knew it would work in this situation as well. It was my way of taking back control of what I could towards achieving a positive outcome.

I performed the routines at a purposeful pace without rushing, so I didn't become anxious or forget to do something I needed to do. When I arrived at the hospital I parked the car purposefully, walked at a regulated pace, kept my head up and smiled. Every day I followed the same routine so I could be in control.

I maintained a confident demeanour and connected with others. Making connections with hospital staff and other patients reminded me to contribute to others and have meaning beyond myself. One such interaction was with a man named Spiros, who was waiting for his radiotherapy treatment. A rotund, jolly Greek man he was always friendly and positive no matter what he talked about. With lightness and fun, he could chat about anything - his life, his wife and family, his diagnosis, and even his short prognosis. He was a real gentleman in how he treated others and exuded delightfulness at every step, despite the enormity of his situation and likelihood that he wouldn't see another Christmas.

I loved these moments, because people like Spiros were so real, open and authentic. He didn't hide anything and talked about the good and the tough moments, including his dreams and aspirations, and how the family would struggle to cope without him. These moments uplifted my spirits. They reinforced there were always others who were doing it tougher, and encouraged me to keep going and be the best version of me, every single day. To do this I applied strategies I had learned from the past to this situation in order to create my new normal.

The 'new normal' was something I needed in my life, and I allowed it to evolve with self-compassion by accepting my limitations, the hardship, the changed abilities, and the lack of being able to push through this. I needed to recognise that I was suffering and accept the situation as it was, which was not an easy feat for me as I was not used to treating myself with compassion. Instead I had always pushed myself to achieve whatever I needed to.

Compassion came slowly by allowing myself to engage in things that would enhance my health and happiness, without self-judgement. For me this was continuing with things that I loved such as being on my bike (even though the distances were short), enjoying the atmosphere of a café, contributing to our business, and interacting with people inside and outside the hospital.

All of these activities were much more limited than before. I wasn't able to cook a complete meal, follow through to the end of a business task, or be around people for too long. The effects of the treatment exhausted me more and more each time, and accumulated. I didn't want to accept this but it was fast becoming my new normal.

Amazingly, I realised my new strategies were actually my old strategies with an adjustment of frequency, intensity and duration. This was about embracing newly revised strategies, bringing through the old successful ones and forging ahead towards accepting the new normal!

Chapter 13

Bouncing Back

When working within the new normal we need to engage the skill of resilience. To me this means adapting by being flexible with thoughts and actions in any situation. People who can keep their cool and adapt positively in the face of trauma, challenges or disaster are described as resilient.

According to Lopez and Snyder (2009), a person who has effective levels of resilience is identified as having the following characteristics: positive self-image; good problem solving skills; the ability to self-regulate; capacity to adapt to many different situations; unwavering faith in one's purpose; a positive outlook on the whole of life; skills and talents that they value about themselves, and are valued by society; and a general acceptance of self. They have the ability to bounce back more quickly, with more clarity and less stress than someone whose resilience is less strongly developed.

Building resilience empowers people to think differently, adapt, change and bounce back in their life at a time of adversity. Being empowered increases one's confidence to deal with the unfamiliar. It allows them to focus on the things that bring out their best because they are more likely to trust themselves and have confidence. They instigate their own innate strengths, use their initiative and allow themselves to be who they really are.

A resilient person does not experience less emotional distress, grief or anxiety than others. They just experience emotions for less time as they have learned not to dwell on them. They recognise the negativity of the moment and make a conscious decision to rapidly shift out of that mental and emotional state.

An example of this may be when two people are made redundant from work. The individual with low levels of resilience may view this as a personal attack and become withdrawn. They focus on the challenges and shortfalls that come with being in this predicament. Their behaviour does them more harm than good because it leaves them feeling unworthy, not good enough and that life is unfair. There is usually a sense that someone or something else is responsible for the situation.

The resilient individual acknowledges they are in unfamiliar territory, states the situation 'as-is', and allows themselves to feel their emotions in that moment. They may feel worried, overwhelmed or nervous, and although the initial impact of the situation may leave them feeling a sense of despair, they will not dwell on those feelings for a long time. Instead they make a conscious decision to focus on opportunities rather than obstacles.

They seek assistance from people, places, or resources and draw on skills and strategies they have used during past struggles, challenges or adversity, and use them again. There is a focus on taking action to transform the situation, with no denial or hiding from it. This is a realistic approach and involves taking control of what can be controlled.

Across the many areas of positive psychology research there are specific personality traits recognised in each individual that set them up to be more resilient than others. The 'Big Five Personality Traits Theory' identified by Robert McCrae and Paul Costa (1987), includes extraversion, openness, agreeableness, conscientiousness and neuroticism.

Extraversion refers to how an individual gains energy. For example, I would make sure I went to a café after treatment to allow myself to shift into feeling more like me. Sitting in a café enjoying a delicious strong skinny piccolo, surrounded by other people enjoying that space, gave me energy.

Someone with a tendency towards introversion would gain their energy from being alone and staying within themselves. Extraversion traits also include being energetic, talkative and assertive. Therefore they are more likely to talk with others, share their responses and ask for help.

Openness identifies the people who seek to learn new things and enjoy new experiences. These individuals have a variety of interests, and are more adventurous and creative in their approach to things they do. This feeds into identifying new strategies to deal with adversity.

Agreeableness includes attributes such as kindness, trust, altruism and other pro-social behaviours such as empathy, helping and standing up for others. The person is more invested in meaning beyond themselves and looks for opportunities to give to others.

Conscientiousness refers to an individual who is good at impulse control (thinks first then responds), is mindful of others and details, is reliable, and finishes tasks they set out to do. They are able to carry through with things without giving up when it gets hard.

Neuroticism entails the concepts of moodiness, sadness and emotional instability. This ignites anxiety, stress and renders them impotent to make decisions.

A resilient person is likely to have high levels of extraversion, openness, agreeableness, conscientiousness and low levels of neuroticism (Oshio, Taku, Hirano, & Saeed, 2018).

There are also key psychological components of resilience. These are self-awareness, courage, adaptability, and flexibility (Lopez & Snyder, 2009). One who possesses these traits is more likely to have or develop higher levels of resilience.

Self-awareness has many different interpretations, but in this context is about understanding personal values, aspirations and responses to various situations. When a person is self-aware, they are able to identify their emotional, mental and physical state. They possess courage and interpret the impact of the sensations they are feeling.

It takes courage to adapt, change and recover from adversity. According to Brené Brown (2015) courage "is a heart word" from the Latin 'cor' and known as "to speak one's mind by telling all one's heart". Having the ability to speak from the heart about who we are and what we are going through, both good and bad, is necessary. When we are able to share from our heart space, we allow ourselves to grow and build resilience even further.

Being adaptable and flexible is having the ability to recover quickly; to remain strong under pressure. One is able to think expansively and transform ideas and concepts into a positive outcome. Researchers are still discussing whether we are born with these traits, or whether they are shaped by environmental factors. Most agree there are components of both. When we recognise the traits we possess and take active steps towards growing and building these further, we set ourselves up for even greater levels of resilience.

These characteristics and key traits need consistent development regardless of the enormity of the challenge. As human beings we tend to cope better when the adverse event is a major one. When something hits us with force, we tend to sit up and take notice of it because we often have no choice to ignore it. It's as if something inside us switches on when the adverse event gets to a point when we can no longer shy away from it. In this moment of urgency we have the option to fold or draw on our strengths to adapt, change and recover.

We are all born with the capacity to be resilient, and anyone can learn strategies, develop habits and acquire techniques to increase resilience if they do the work. Resilience does not just appear after experiencing trauma or pain. It is not an endpoint. Building resilience occurs before, during and after adverse events and is fluid and dynamic.

George Bonanno (Professor of Clinical Psychology at Columbia University) emphasises that perception is a central element of resilience (2004). Every event that elicits an emotion has the potential to be traumatic, depending on the perception of the person experiencing it. We can perceive an event as either being traumatic, or an opportunity to learn and grow.

Bonanno explains that if you take something as terrible as the surprising death of a close friend you might be distraught, but if you can find a way to construe that event as filled with meaning, then it can lead to greater awareness or closer connections (2004). For example, you may discover a greater understanding of a certain disease or develop closer ties with a community of people. The event can then be reinterpreted as something other than trauma.

I recall the moment I received a phone call letting me know that a friend had died unexpectedly. I was in shock to think that such a thing could happen to her. She was a strong, high-achieving person. A high-ranking police officer, contributing to and changing the lives of many individuals and communities, and living her life to the fullest - mentally, physically, and emotionally. One day it all became too much and she took her own life. A couple of days after hearing this sad news I learned she also had a debilitating type of arthritis and would have soon needed to be in a wheelchair. There is no way to know the full story as to why Brigitte suicided, but she did. A letter to her parents explained that she did not want to be a cripple, and had run out of puff.

As I processed the devastating loss of such an amazing woman, I was able to attribute meaning to it so it was not traumatic for me. It was very sad, shocking and devastating, but not traumatic. This was someone who had run the entire 805km El Camino trail, completed several Ironman events including Hawaii and Mexico, cycled across the South Island of New Zealand with her husband for fun, went to the gym most days of her adult life (no matter what), and was continually on-the-go changing people's lives.

I understood that if she could not be this energetic person and continue her lifestyle the way she wanted, she would lose her identity and her ability to be independent and in control. She could not face being in a wheelchair and having disability and impairment as her identity.

In the process of writing this book, I was in touch with Brigitte's husband again because I wanted to pay my respects to them both. He gifted me these words as a tribute to the amazing things she accomplished:

"Brigitte was and still is an amazing woman to me. Every family celebration we still charge a glass and remember the amazing times and her achievements. [I am] proud that Brigitte has put processes in place to care for our most vulnerable [people] in our community (regardless of gender or race)! Brigitte's dedication to New Zealand (albeit tragedies) was strong, never wavered. [She was involved in] the Cave Creek disaster, ODARA [Ontario Domestic Assault Assessment processes], the Pike River Mine disaster, the Christchurch earthquake, she could not give anymore. Okay, I could go on and on, [I] still love her and always will!"

Bonanno states that an individual's experience is not inherent in the event; it resides in the event's psychological construct. That is, our understanding and the meaning we attribute to the event takes away the overwhelm of emotion and makes sense of a situation; looking at the what and why around the event, rather than getting caught up directly in the emotion.

By attributing a psychological response, I can still make a connection with Brigitte, her pain, her situation, and her decision. I don't have to like or agree with it, but I can begin to make sense of it. In our interpretation and conceptualisation of an event we either assign trauma to it or not.

Having the ability to consciously engage our resilience creates a remarkable space for us to connect with a person or situation with meaning and purpose. Resilience is like a muscle, the same as the muscles in our body; we must deliberately and consistently train to strengthen our resilience for the purpose we desire. When an individual consciously practises resiliency skills in everyday life, they develop the strength, flexibility and capability of their resilience muscle to work when required.

Each outcome we desire has a different training program. We cannot work blindly and hope to achieve the desired goal. We must work with a purposeful intention, and engage the correct training program to master the outcome or goal we desire. Yes, there will be days when we feel tired, and moments within the workout when we feel like we cannot keep going.

Resilience is not a one-time job. It takes diligence and consistency. As we master each small step along the way we gain more and more strength and flexibility in our resilience muscle. We must work to endure the uncomfortable moments of the unknown. We need to do the heavy lifting and repetitions to make the gains. It is something we must work at habitually, invest in and develop over our entire lifetime.

The way I engaged my resilience muscle each day to be my best and participate in tasks, was to stick wholeheartedly to the routines that worked for me. Each day I would check in with myself and notice how I was feeling (mentally, physically, and emotionally) and then take actions accordingly. I had unwavering faith that things would work out, and as long as I kept doing what kept me at my best, then it would work. This was not about being careless or stupid, but engaging my intellect, my experience and all of my strengths to be consistent with everything I did.

I didn't just get up every day and randomly select something to do. I purposefully evoked my resilience and applied this to continue learning what would work for me. This included identifying possibilities, researching alternative methods, and integrating all of these components into my personal understanding of my strengths and abilities.

Tayyab Rashid, a Clinical Psychologist in Positive Psychology, along with Seligman identified that engaging in an intentional habitual practice to strengthen resilience reduces stress, increases healthy mental function, strengthens fulfilling relationships, and creates a meaningful life (2019).

Rashid states that purposefully identifying the positives in life like our strengths, talents and skills, while also engaging in daily gratitude, intensifies our resilience muscle. We also know that where our focus and attention goes, our energy flows. If an individual focuses on weaknesses, deficits or challenges they are likely to get stuck in that negative thought pattern, which becomes their emphasis for all thoughts and actions. With a negative thought pattern they will have difficulty instigating their resilience muscle, and will remain pessimistic.

We have the choice of tapping into the positive aspects of our life and engaging optimism. When we shift our mindset towards positives, we are aware of what we *do* have rather than what we *don't* have. What we *can* do rather than what we *can't* do. Our vibe becomes more upbeat, our emotional state is less angry, less stressed, less frustrated, and we become genuinely happier about ourselves and our life.

During this entire journey throughout my diagnosis, treatment and recovery, I have focused on what strengths I could bring to the experience to maintain a positive mindset. I engaged daily in gratitude, often up to two or three times a day at home with Elizabeth, and in general conversations with people I encountered. I made sure I presented the best version of myself every day throughout treatment and check-ups. I took my strengths with me to each visit and intentionally focused on what was going well. This boosted my mental functioning and strengthened my resilience muscle even further.

"While it's not possible to eliminate all setbacks and adversity people face in life, it is achievable to enhance the use of our strengths and learn new skills to deal with the challenges that life throws our way".

The concept of positive emotions and how they affect resilience was explored by Michele Tugade (Professor of Psychological Science at Vassar College) and Barbara Fredrickson (2007). For an individual to bounce back after trauma or setback it is vital to engage in positive emotions.

This was further researched by Laura Kiken (Professor at Kent University) and Barbara Fredrickson (2017) who identified that when individuals engage in daily positive emotions they bounce back faster from negative events and daily stress. Kiken and Fredrickson point out that positive emotions literally change the way we see things (2017). They affect visual attention (what we see) as well as our perception (how we interpret what we see).

For example, we may view the walk to work as filled with things that are broken or drab, or we may 'see' the tree, the weed flower, and the brightly coloured graffiti. When individuals regularly experience positive emotions their agency (ability to achieve an intended goal) is increased. Positive emotions speed up our psychological recovery time to negative events, and decrease the overall harm that an adverse event might cause. Purposefully initiating a positive mood increases our pain tolerance and decreases physiological recovery time. The key is to maintain and strengthen our resilience muscle, to engage in daily practices that elicit positive emotions.

The individual who has worked on their resilience muscle consistently is more likely to see themselves as a survivor, and may even thrive in the face of adversity. They will take control of their thoughts, feelings and actions with the intention of maintaining the best version of themselves, and recover quickly. Whereas the individual who has a low level of resilience will struggle with adversity and setbacks, and remain stuck in negative emotions and thinking. They often become a victim within the circumstance, perceive they have little control of their life, blame others and are unable to help themselves.

Individuals with low levels of resilience engage regularly in negative self-talk. This is where our internal dialogue continues incessantly on repeat mode. Self-talk is a combination of unconscious beliefs and biases and our conscious thoughts. We have around 60,000 thoughts a day and we can choose what to focus on. When individuals with a low level of resilience believe they are a victim, this perpetuates the focus on negative self-talk and perceptions.

For example, in this instance, much of the internal dialogue and vocalised chatter may be: "Life is unfair"; "Everybody else knows what to do except me"; "They obviously don't think much of me"; "They don't trust me"; "I'm useless"; "I can't do that"; "This always happens to me". Persisting with this negative self-talk creates a perpetual negative spiral and takes a toll on our emotional state, weakening our ability to bounce back. If we believe this to be our truth we render ourselves powerless, cement our negative view of the world, and diminish our resilience.

Amrisha Vaish (Associate Professor at Max Planck Institute for Evolutionary Anthropology) and colleagues stated, "not all emotions are created equal" with ample evidence to demonstrate the negativity bias in human beings (Vaish, Grossmann, & Woodward, 2008). This suggests that human beings are pre-disposed to connecting with negative information and negative self-talk. This highlights that we actually focus on and hear the negative as the dominating voice which causes us to respond more strongly to negative stimuli.

Think of it this way. If we receive the same amount of positive and negative input, our response to the negative input is much greater. When we give this negativity more focus it becomes the centre of our attention. The more attention and focus we give it, the more it stays with us. This is a cyclical challenge of negativity, hopelessness and apathy.

Whereas if we regularly engage in positive self-talk, it boosts our optimism, hope, and joy. It changes the chemicals and structure of our cells. This positive internal dialogue is not used to deceive ourselves or cover up something that may harm us. It is the truth. Positive self-talk is recognising the truth within ourselves, the situation and the environment that we are in.

Christopher Carr, the Sport Performance Psychologist from St Vincent Sports Performance in Indianapolis, uses these principles when working with international sports teams in the USA (2006). He uses positive self-talk to boost emotions, confidence and self-worth, which ultimately impacts performance. When we use positive self-talk that is relevant to the situation, it results in an emotional experience of relaxation, calm and centredness, allowing us to perform at our best with the least amount of emotional and physical effort.

The way I kept on top of my self-talk with the least amount of effort possible, was to begin the day with a few wise positive words to myself. Firstly, it was "yes, I'm here and I get to have another awesome day". It wasn't that I didn't know if I would wake up or not. It did make me smile and got me thinking about myself, taking control of what I *could* do and what I *did* have in my life at that current point in time.

I engaged and recognised the positive things I heard, saw and felt each day on my way to treatment, during treatment, at the check-ups and after treatment. I would smell the amazing eucalyptus trees as I walked into the hospital grounds and repeatedly think positive thoughts. I would smile at people and think something positive about them, whether it was what they were wearing or how they interacted with me. It was the truth. It was not a cover up or lie. It was not pretence. I consciously engaged in positive thoughts, even when I was sitting in the waiting room for what seemed like forever. I would notice what was beyond the window, or the bright colour of something, or what I would do after treatment.

The way to take back control of our thoughts and emotional state is by engaging in positive psychological techniques. These proven Positive Psychology techniques include practising daily mindfulness and/or meditation. Dr Craig Hassed, a general practitioner and lecturer on mindfulness at Monash University, describes mindfulness as a form of meditation and way of living (2008). He states that it's not about sitting in a chair and practising mindfulness or meditation for five minutes a day. It's about being attentive, present and engaged, with an open and accepting attitude to all our daily events.

Mindfulness is focused on attention regulation, noticing where our attention and thoughts are, and gently bringing them back to the present.

Hassed describes this as:

1) Knowing where our attention is
2) Prioritising where it needs to be
3) Moving our attention to go 'there' and stay there.

Often we are distracted, may not have heard a conversation, did not taste a mouthful of dinner, or comprehended anything we were reading. Many times we are what is called 'away with the fairies'.

Our attention is on a different moment (either past or future) from the current one. We therefore need to prioritise the present moment, bring ourselves back to it and engage in it fully for us to give our best. Once we are conscious of where our attention needs to be, the challenge is then to move it over and keep it there. This is a skill that requires repetition in order to be harnessed and magnified.

When we are fully engaged in what we are doing, hearing, seeing and smelling in the present moment, our performance increases. We hear more, see more, feel more, taste more, smell more. Practising mindfulness has been shown to reduce stress, change gene expression in only four days (which changes our health status), lengthen our telomeres (that determine longevity of life), boost our immune system, and enable us to live a longer, happier life.

I practise mindfulness and meditation by engaging all my senses while doing guided meditations. I have trained myself over the years to be totally in the moment. Part of this comes from my hockey training, and the rest has been honed over recent years. When I have my morning coffee I use a cup without a handle. I create a ritual around the grinding of the beans, the measuring of the water, the stirring of the coffee with a special wooden spatula from New Zealand, and then I wait.

I look out the window at something bigger than me such as a tree or the sky. I wait for exactly four minutes before I pour that liquid gold into my cup. Seeing it, smelling it, hearing it. I watch the MCT oil that I add to the cup dance on the top, and know that is extra added goodness for my health. Then comes the moment of anticipation. The first mouthful. A moment when I pause with the cup near my mouth. I smell the intensified aroma, feel the warmth of the cup in my hand, and then I taste. I savour this moment – the first mouthful of the cup. The moment of sheer joy and oneness with myself, the environment and the task I am engaged in is pure bliss.

I also conduct this mindful ritual in other areas of my life. All the usual tasks that are embedded in the 'normal' day to day experiences of life, including cleaning my teeth, doing a work out, and eating my meals. I have attributed meaning to each moment, task, and time, which gets me through the day and refreshes me so that I keep going no matter what situation or setback I may be facing. These moments during the day are not massive chunks of time. The time it takes to make a French press coffee is still the same. The time it takes to brush my teeth is still the same. The time it takes to do a workout is the same. There is no added time pressure; it is a purposeful intention to be in the moment.

As for meditation, this is a journey I am still on. A technique that I am practising and building into a habit to find what works for me in terms of music, voice, emphasis, and style. We can embrace meditation tools and strategies that others have already forged. We do not need to create them ourselves when we are learning the practice. We can make our lives better by embedding these habits into our routine. They make us stronger, empower us to thrive and give us the fuel to carry on another day.

There is a great deal of evidence surrounding the concept that individuals who engage in meditation or mindfulness develop a stronger sense of purpose in their life. Jay Shetty, former monk, author and motivational speaker, explains that at its root purpose meditation serves to help with self-awareness, break down the different identities we create for ourselves, and enables us to reveal our true self.

He describes the process of meditation and mindfulness as "uncovering and accepting all of self - the good, the bad and the ugly". We need to recognise all of self before we can be our true self and live our purpose fully by not compartmentalising our roles or beliefs to match a certain situation. We need to be able to sit in stillness and be with ourselves. Without judgement, without critique we also need to be able to ask ourselves the tough questions, learn the tricks of our mind, and turn these around when required. Meditation and mindfulness allow us to create the space in our mind to discover our true self, determine the meaning beyond ourselves and uncover our true purpose.

Ed Diener's extensive research on the science of wellbeing has found that people with a strong sense of purpose are better able to handle the ups and downs of life and to keep getting up despite setbacks, to persevere and continue moving forward. This strong sense of life purpose buffers the day-to-day challenges and augments resilience in the individual. This purpose provides motivation and direction for an individual to be the captain of their own ship and keep going no matter what.

Research completed by Stacey Schaefer and colleagues (2013) at the University of Leicester has identified that having a strong sense of purpose in life enables individuals to reframe stressful situations and deal with adversity more productively and quickly. This links strongly back to the notion of PERMA (discussed earlier in this book), where M stands for meaning beyond self. Purpose and meaning are therefore vital constructs to leading a long, happy, healthy and satisfying life.

Dan Buettner, founder of Blue Zones, an organisation researching the world's longest-lived cultures, confirms that meaning is one of the essentials to living a long and happy life (2010). Buettner and colleagues identified geographical regions which are home to some of the world's healthiest and oldest people including Ikaria, Greece; Loma Linda, California; Sardinia, Italy; Okinawa, Japan; and Nicoya, Costa Rica. These Blue Zones are classified by the high number of healthy centenarians living there. Within these regions they discovered the main reason for longevity of women in Okinawa was the strong sense of meaning they had in their lives. This included being healthy, connecting and contributing to others in their community, and across generations.

Okinawans are known for pursuing *ikigai* – a Japanese concept meaning 'a reason for being'. This concept is seen as the convergence of four primary elements:
1) What you love (your passion)
2) What the world needs (your mission)
3) What you are good at (your vocation)
4) What you can get paid for (your profession).

Discovering your own *ikigai* is said to bring fulfillment, happiness and makes you live longer.

According to Buettner, the concept of *ikigai* is not exclusive to Okinawans (2010). He identified that in all four blue zones there were people living long lives using this concept. The secret to *ikigai* is not to focus on one element, but to utilise all four. Most people do not achieve an end point in *ikigai*. The whole essence of *ikigai* is to progress closer to the intersectionality of the four elements. It is in the seeking of such a state that one discovers the next level of purpose towards a clearly defined pathway to pursuing their passion, no matter what. They never give up, and have the ability to get back on track even when everything is stacked against them. Everyone can experience *ikigai,* even in the hardest of times, by taking even the smallest of steps forward with purpose.

Chapter 14

Authentic Resilience

Adversity can be transformed into advantage. However, for this transformative growth to occur, we must first be catapulted out of our usual mental, physical, emotional and spiritual state into unknown turmoil with curiosity and openness. Not an easy task to contemplate when your life is feeling out of control. It is easier to shift back into the known where it's comfortable and stay the same as before, albeit a low resilience state, and bounce back to previous levels of performance.

However, there is an additional level of resilience where we can bounce forward to a different time and space. This demonstrates the ability to learn from our experiences, set an optimistic mindset, and take action forward. When we are able to do this, we come through situations with more ease, less hurt, and less stress. Although we have more tools and strategies in our toolbox, our life approach and ethos may remain the same. Even though we have high levels of resilience at this stage, we may not experience the next level of resilience known as post-traumatic growth.

Tedeschi and colleagues (1996) originally describe the concept of Post-Traumatic Growth (PTG) as the point at which someone is rocked to their core within a trauma. They have had their fundamental beliefs extensively challenged and chosen to change. They have developed a different appreciation for life, re-evaluated their purpose and meaning, and created a self-promise to live a meaningful life. They experience personal advancement due to the tumultuous psychological struggle of the trauma.

The individual who experiences PTG is able to see a pathway forward for themselves that is very different to what once was. They have clarity, certainty and fulfillment in their life at a much higher level than before the trauma. They cope with and deal with challenges in a positive light and are no longer stuck in their story or past events. The individual has a deeper understanding of themselves and how to live their life going forward. Instead of turning to their logical response, they turn to their heart. They turn to their essence of being, and question their identity, their beliefs and what they stand for. They question what is truly important to them in that moment forward and find resolution on how to live life. The person will never be the same again.

Not everyone experiences this positive growth as a result of trauma. Even though an individual may often display high levels of resilience, it is not a given that they will experience post traumatic growth. If the individual is focused on returning to their pre-trauma routines and habits, then that is the threshold they will attain. They will not see a way of living beyond their current status of 'just getting by'. If the individual allows their fear of a new normal to control them, they will go back to how it was before.

An individual who experiences PTG may still experience grief, anxiety, anger and negative thoughts, but these do not take over their life or the majority of their thoughts. Tedeschi estimates that only one half to two thirds of people experience PTG after trauma. It depends on the type of trauma, the individual's personal circumstances, the timing of how far through the journey the individual is, and how they define their life. He also states that a precursor to developing PTG is that the individual is open to reconsidering their belief systems.

Tedeschi and colleagues have also identified two traits in people most likely to experience PTG, which are openness and extraversion. People who are open to new ideas and embrace new ways of doing life are more likely to question and re-assess their personal beliefs. This allows them to see obstacles as opportunities.

A person displaying extraversion will be active in their response to the trauma. They will seek out connections with others and share their thoughts and feelings rather than bottle them up. Tedeschi and colleagues noted in their research that more women than men experience PTG, because women are more inclined to be open, share their experiences, and connect with others on a deeper level than men.

Here are two remarkable stories and examples of people who developed Post Traumatic Growth and made an impact on my life.

Gill Hicks (AM, MBE, FRSA)

Coming back from the dead and literally being labelled as 'one unknown' was not how Gill Hicks, founder of the London based M.A.D. for Peace organisation, ever saw her life. Gill tells her story as a survivor of the July 7, 2005 London bombings. She was on her way to work in London, on the Tube. Little did she or the other people in that carriage know their life was about to change in an instant. The bomb blast was beyond her comprehension. The carriage plummeted into darkness and the terrorist attack left her without legs and fighting for life. It also caused damage to her hearing, lungs and vocal cords.

As Gill lay in the wreckage of the carriage with dead bodies around her, she made an instant decision. If she was somehow able to survive this horrific ordeal, then she would 'make the rest of her life count'. She fought the urge to close her eyes because she knew if she did, she would certainly die. Instead she lowered her breathing rate, elevated her thighs, tied her scarf around her legs as a tourniquet to stop the bleeding, and did all she could to survive. All the while she took her turn with other survivors to repeat a roll call: 'I am Gill... I'm here... I'm alive'. It was one whole hour later before she felt the safe touch of her rescuers.

Gill's ability to make a decision to choose life over giving up was the first sign of being rocked to her core. Her foundational beliefs of life were challenged in that moment. She chose to find meaning beyond herself. She found an appreciation for her life and in that instant, Gill decided to do everything she could to survive. When she was through the moment of just surviving, she then decided to thrive.

Still to this day Gill talks about experiencing the psychological, emotional and physical trauma of that day. However, she does not dwell on the horrific ordeal and remain in the past. She finds possibilities in each new day. She has strong meaningful connections with her family and friends. Since that experience in July 2005 she has a new-found appreciation for life. She is now devoted to Making A Difference (M.A.D.) throughout the world and inspiring people to rise above trauma and adversity.

Viktor E Frankl (MD, PhD)

Viktor E. Frankl, the Austrian psychiatrist, author of 'Man's Search for Meaning', and founder of the field of Logotherapy, spent three torturous years in concentration camps during the Second World War (1992). In his writings, he said that he was robbed of everything he had as a human being except the ability to find meaning in the suffering. The atrocities he experienced and observed did not break his spirit. He worked out how to rise above his current situation and chose an attitude of hope and optimism.

Through the many extreme and vicious acts that were inflicted on Frankl in various camps, he maintained the ability to find meaning in the suffering. Even in the depths of torture, suffering and humiliation, Frankl decided to suffer bravely because it gave him a reason and a purpose each day. He writes about the differences between the prisoners who were able to wake up each day with purpose, and those who could not. The latter did not survive. How did anyone have a choice within such inhospitable circumstances?

As Frankl put it, "When we are no longer able to change a situation, we are challenged to change ourselves" (1992, p112). The prisoners who changed their mindset and found meaning whilst enduring the horrors of war, were far more resilient than those who did not. The one thing Frankl did differently from those without hope and optimism was he did not dwell on the trauma or allow it to consume him.

The decision to find meaning in the moment, to find meaning in the suffering was a key to dealing with the mental, physical and emotional trauma. Frankl states that the last of the human freedoms cannot be taken from us – our attitude. "What alone remains is the last of human freedoms … the ability to choose one's attitude in a given set of circumstances" (1992, p65-68).

The way we think about any given situation is within our control. Frankl spoke of how he held onto his freedom of choice each day by finding moments of joy in the small things, such as the sunrise, or being the lucky one to get the 4-5 peas in the so-called soup that was served. He would notice the joy in the moment when one of his fellow prisoners gave another a small piece of hidden bread. He savoured these small moments of joy.

He held onto his belief that he would have a life beyond the concentration camps, with optimism and hope. If we choose to view a situation with hope and optimism, and allow ourselves to experience our full spectrum of emotions, then we too can find meaning and growth in the situation. Frankl also experienced many times of grief, despondency and abhorrence but chose not to let them determine his outcome.

These two real life stories have much in common. The point at which Gill Hicks and Viktor Frankl made a deliberate decision to choose life was when they were rocked to the core, and their fundamental beliefs were severely challenged. Gill decided that she would do everything within her control to save herself mentally, physically and emotionally and then make the rest of her life count.

Viktor made the decision to find meaning in the suffering and control the only thing he could control at that point, his attitude. Mentally, physically and emotionally they were both stretched and confronted beyond comprehension. Yet amongst all their horrifying experiences they both made the decision that had an extraordinary impact on the rest of their lives. This defining juncture is where they tapped into their hope, self-efficacy, resilience and optimism (H.E.R.O.).

This is what I aimed to do during this time of diagnosis and treatment, and continue to do today and every day of my precious life.

Developing H.E.R.O.

An individual who views extreme challenges with **H**ope (seeing present and future moments with positive emotion), is able to dig deep into their psychological resources and construct a pathway forward. This is known as pathway thinking. The second part of hope is when the individual follows through on their initial thoughts, takes action and builds confidence in their ability to keep going. This is known as agency thinking, the ability to view challenging situations with hope, anticipate obstacles and unknowns along the way, and still expect to attain their goal. These people take persistent action, even when the going gets tough, because they tap into their reason, purpose, and drive for life.

This can be reaffirmed by a statement or mantra that one adheres to. The mantra that I have always used from a young age is, "there is always a way". I purposefully used this before, during and after treatment. I needed to believe in the medical team to do their part and also believe in myself that I could do it because there was a way.

To maintain a belief in oneself to achieve a successful outcome requires a high level of **Efficacy** (confidence). The higher our efficacy we have in self (self-efficacy), the harder we will work to achieve our goals. When we truly believe in ourselves, we are more likely to be successful. Whereas an individual who has a low level of self-efficacy is unlikely to reach their goals. Self-efficacy can be increased by being open to new ideas and seeing obstacles as opportunities. Even in the most challenging situations, an individual with high self-efficacy will engage their curiosity to learn from the situation and strengthen their resolve.

The notion of **Resilience** within psychological capital is to bounce back from challenges, risks and trauma. When things go wrong in life, our resilience enables us to get back up, keep going and return to our normal usual functioning. As we discussed earlier, resilience is the ability to adapt and problem solve in the midst of challenge or trauma. We all experience some form of rejection, challenge or trauma in life. But the difference between those who give up and those who keep going is not about the degree of hardship they endured, but the ability to bounce back and go again.

Optimism (the belief that an outcome will be favourable) is an essential characteristic to cope with life's challenges. An optimist believes that things will go well now, in the future when (not if) the next challenge strikes. The optimist will remind themselves of the lessons and benefits they have received from previous and current situations. They accept the reality of the adversity faster than pessimists because they do not ruminate on the trauma.

Optimists are able to stop themselves being caught up in the negative spiral of hopelessness. Even though they still experience distress, grief and pain, they adapt quickly to situations by reinterpreting the situation with a positive mindset. The difference between a pessimist (feeling hopeless) and an optimist (feeling hopeful) is that they choose to reframe the event and shift their attention and thoughts to an adaptive process.

An individual with high levels of psychological capital (H.E.R.O.) is healthier mentally, physically and emotionally. When we boost one pillar of psychological capital there is a positive ripple effect across the other pillars. Individuals with a high overall psychological capital believe they can control their future and that things will work out well in the end. When facing adversity they are able to adapt quickly, instigate a change of focus, and maintain their future-orientated approach.

As I neared the end of treatment, I made a conscious decision to focus on how I would 'do life' going forward. I invested a great deal of time and effort into thinking, planning, setting up and creating an environment that would have me at my best each day. I was internally driven to maintain high levels of hope and optimism. Every single day I called on my resilience to keep me going. My medical team could not provide me with a definitive answer of being cancer free; friends could not support me in this endeavour, I had to do it for myself. I knew that the more belief I had in myself, the better off I would be. I was still choosing life.

As the treatment chapter of my life came to a close I headed towards changes once again in my now familiar daily routines. I had to once again choose how I would keep rising, mentally, physically and emotionally, out of this ordeal. I likened it to the end of any sporting event or training routine. It's one small part of the bigger picture. It's an intersection where you can choose to either turn left or right. This is a phase that generates many unknowns. It is also a point that opens up a plethora of opportunities.

Each Wednesday I had a regular appointment with my Radiation Oncologist which took extra conviction to approach with optimism. Each time I visited, part of me was emotionally propelled back into the same feeling of being in limbo. I was scared of not knowing what would happen next. I was dealing with the cumulative physical effects of the treatment, and asked myself a multitude of questions. How did I know if the treatment worked? When would I know if it did work? What could I do to make sure I didn't get worse? As the appointments began to be spaced out, I believed that I was no longer controlled by cancer and its many facets of treatments, appointments, preparation and side effects. I was controlled by me.

A new phase was beginning. My new normal was changing again. I needed to rediscover how to set myself up in the morning to be the best version of myself. I wouldn't see my 'team mates' every day, so who could I chat with that would understand what I was going through? Who were my new team mates? How do I know if I'm doing 'life' right, given my diagnosis? This was all new again and I didn't have anything to gauge life against. I hadn't been here before. I didn't know what to think, what emotional state to be in, and I certainly didn't know what to do.

Again, I needed to tell myself to shut up and listen, get on top of my emotions, and tune in to my body and mind so I could thrive. I had to consciously shift my mindset into another phase of coping, dig deep into my toolkit and haul out more of my knowledge, understanding and expertise. I needed to instigate yet another strategy that could propel me from this place of unknown to a place of assurance. I had to remember that I did know what to think, I did know what emotional state would serve me, and I did know what actions I needed to take to be at my best. I had done this all before in similar situations. Yes, this one was new, but I had been challenged before and pushed through mentally, physically and emotionally to achieve success.

I totally believed I would be all right and would get through this horrifying ordeal, fundamentally believing I would be even better than I was prior to the diagnosis. I also believed I would learn things about others and myself that I had never known before.

Throughout this ordeal, I was regularly thrust outside my comfort zone. Sometimes it was my choice to step outside my comfort zone, and other times it was a matter of trusting the process and believing that my medical team had my best interests at heart. Embarking on what was yet another unknown was another one of those moments to trust the process, trust myself and trust the universe that it would all work out perfectly.

Your limitless possibilities...

1) Set yourself purposeful routines
   - Smile when you wake in the morning
   - Perform your routines at a purposeful pace
2) Create meaningful connections with others
   - Identify the positives in the moments to begin the connection

- Be open with yourself and others
3) Continue to cultivate your resilience muscle
   - Enhance your self-awareness
   - Embrace adaptability and flexibility of thought
4) Purposefully begin your day with intention
   - Set your intention for the day
   - Follow through with action on this intention
5) Tap into your self-talk
   - Engage in optimistic self-talk to boost hope and joy
6) Be fully present in your activities
   - Tune all your senses into your tasks and activities
   - Practice meditation/mindfulness
7) Life is dynamic and fluid, maneuver with it!

THE EMPOWERMENT

* * *

Affirmation: "I am bigger than my circumstances"

Chapter 15

Second Chances

As I head beyond four-years post diagnosis, I pause and recognise that I am still learning new things about myself. New things about life and how to live in the present moment, because this is the only thing we truly have. The now! Yes, I do look forward to the future and I intentionally plan that too, but I don't stay focused on it at the expense of the now. I look forward to things being even more amazing than they are right now, and plan what, where and how life will be further down the track. I also plan forward in our business, so we can empower even more clients.

I plan to grow wiser, healthier, and absolutely plan on being here for a very long time to come. I have work to do, gifts to share, fun to experience, changes to make and a whole lot of inspiration and influence to spread around.

My desire is to live each and every day on purpose! Not squandering opportunities, resources or time, but choosing to live a life full of intention, driven towards my purpose. I am completely aware that how I interact, inspire and influence people has gone to a much higher level since that moment of diagnosis. I am committed to creating and maintaining deeper connections with people, and to bringing the best version of myself forward every single day. No matter what.

I embrace the fact that I have been given a second chance. A wakeup call and an opportunity to do life differently. It's not the journey I would have chosen for myself or wished on anyone else, however, I do believe experiencing a traumatic event, setback or major change in one's life, can definitely be a defining moment. If we let it.

At the time of diagnosis and any other setback since, I decided I would always give life my best shot. This means learning more about my strengths, knowing myself in greater depth, and purposefully selecting what truly serves me. When I do what aligns with my purpose, the better my life is, the deeper connections I have, and the more I can serve others. During this time I also decided I would only let the people who support, challenge and stretch me into my team. I do life differently.

For me, doing life differently means living each day with a purpose and meaning beyond myself. That bigger 'thing' that is linked to the reason I am here. This is no accident; I have a purpose for being here on this planet at this time. Having a purpose in life is not about being busy all the time, and not about being dictated to or being a people pleaser. It's about being laser-focused on the reason I am here. It's about keeping myself powerful, Authentic and resilient so I can be the most magnificent version of me.

Now, being powerful is not coming from a place of ego, authoritarianism or having power over people. It is about being confident and self-accepting, aware of my shadow self, embracing all the parts of me, and being in the best state possible mentally, physically, emotionally and spiritually. When I am in this powerful state and following my true purpose, I can serve those who are ready to hear my message.

My purpose is to have an element of fun in everything I do and inspire people to be the best versions of themselves, every single day, no matter what.

You may ask how does one find their purpose as there are many different ways to discover this. Each person needs to discover their own specific purpose, meaning or 'why' in life. It is not something others can determine for you. If you ask Google 'how do I find my purpose?' (as I did on the day I was writing this part) you will find more than 1,700,000,000 results. You'd think it would be easy to work out your purpose and follow through with one of these billion ways. Yet generally speaking, most humans amble through life, with very little or no purpose at all.

Doing life without a purpose is like a leaf just blowing in the wind. Like a small stick being tossed in an ocean of waves. It feels like someone has the remote control to you and your life where you are at the mercy of those around you, ambling through life aimlessly, believing you have no say in what happens to you. But your life is a choice, and you get to choose your response to life every single moment of every day.

As Jim Carrey said in his commencement speech in 2014 to the graduates at Maharishi University of Management in Iowa, "When I say life doesn't happen to you, it happens for you, I really don't know if that's true. I'm just making a conscious choice to perceive challenges as something beneficial so that I can deal with them in the most productive way". This notion that life happens *for* you, is remarkably powerful if you choose to perceive it in this way. You have the remote, you get to choose!

Many people spend their life thinking that everything is happening *to* them, as they go through the years wildly riding the next wave of whatever happens *to* them. The next drama, the next incident, the next illness, the next… They only notice or react after things have happened, or when they go wrong. They get caught up in the negativity and distress of the situation. They are reactive and spend their time merely responding to situations and not planning, preparing or regulating themselves for success. Doing life in this way is exhausting and uncomfortable.

If we align our thinking to "life happens *for* us rather than *to* us" as Jim Carrey points out, then we can live life in a purposeful and powerful way. With this optimistic view on life, we will experience those situations that challenge us and push us to our limits in such a way that we are open to receiving the learning. When we recognise these challenging moments as a lesson, an opportunity that is beneficial, then we will grow and evolve.

Perceiving our circumstances as a possibility rather than an edict, allows us to become a better person. We become the person who is bigger than our circumstances. The person who is not controlled by external situations, people or environments, but one whose life happens *for* them. We become the victor and learn how to control the controllable. We stand up for what we believe in and take action on those things that serve us well. We step out with meaning and intention to follow our purpose and take control of our own life. We do this through reframing our thought processes, accepting the reality, and making decisions that propel us forward with momentum.

For this forward momentum to occur we must live not only intentionally, but also consciously. Living consciously is choosing to participate in each and every moment, being *present*. Engaging all of our senses, taking back control, thinking about and making purposeful decisions. When we live consciously, we set ourselves up to be our best version in that moment. This lessens the time spent ruminating on negative thoughts and allows us the space and presence to select thoughts and actions that not only serve us well, but contribute to others beyond ourselves.

Having a purpose, a 'why', or a quest, provides the drive and platform to overcome any obstacle. Viktor Frankl quotes the philosopher Friedrich Nietzsche "he who has a why to live, can bear almost any how" (1992, p9). Powerful words! Our purpose is the 'thing' that reminds us which direction we are heading, why we are heading there, who we are to 'be', and how we are to 'do' life.

When we follow our pathway, stay true to our purpose and understand our why, we are happier, healthier and have much deeper connections with ourself and others. Living life in alignment with our purpose or why, creates a situation where life makes sense. We have a reason for being here. We matter in the world and feel a sense of value and worth.

Napoleon Hill (author of 'Think and Grow Rich') once said, "There is one quality that one must possess to win, and that is definiteness of purpose, the knowledge of what one wants, and a burning desire to possess it" (1987, p45). This is not about likening ourselves to others, or having a burning desire to be better than everyone else. It means we must live life with a desire to fulfill our purpose, to take action and go after it.

To get what you want in life you must decide to move towards what is going to serve you as your highest self. The process of working towards your higher self is self-actualisation and moving towards attaining your highest potential. This is about the journey, the waiting, the moving, the pauses, and the action. It will not happen without ACTION. It is vital to take MASSIVE intentional action because our human mind naturally wants to keep us safe, hold us back, or demand we take tiny, secure steps.

This is how we have kept safe in the past. However, when we take massive action we disrupt the brain's logical thinking processes, the limitations, and the excuses. We rewire our neurology and instigate bigger leaps in the direction of our purpose. The most successful people in the world (and I'm not just talking about money wealth, but life wealth – who they BE!), have a definite focused direction, a strong sense of purpose and take intentional massive action on a consistent basis, no matter what!

When you work intentionally and consciously on taking massive action towards being your highest self, you will experience a stronger sense of purpose that fuels your internal drive, and propels you forward with certainty. I am still challenged by this in my life each day, and want to share one last story with you.

Chapter 16

Coffee, Chemo and Cookies

H ere I was complaining about running out of coffee beans. As you know by now, this is part of my morning ritual of gratitude. Savouring a coffee moment is linked to my purpose and is one of my priorities in life. It is how I take moments in my day to fill up my tank, and it adds to my priorities of maintaining strong connections with people and inspiring them to reach higher levels of greatness. I have my routine of a coffee moment before any coaching or training session. I slow down, connect with myself in a mindful way, instigate all my senses, and create a moment of flow.

I was getting incredibly frustrated at myself and everyone else in the world for leaving it until the last minute to re-order. My massive intentional action was directed at acquiring the best possible delicious coffee beans in the shortest possible timeframe.

Here we were, in stage four lockdown (during the Covid-19 Pandemic), in Melbourne, Australia. At the time we were the most restricted city in the world, unable to go further than 5 kilometres for only one hour, with night-time curfews in place. I was thinking of all the possible options I could employ to get the beans I liked within these restrictions, in case the favourite beans that I'd ordered didn't get here in time.

I was totally consumed by the need for coffee beans and the impact it would cause me if those beans did not arrive before the current supply ran out. I'm sure you can feel my pain and frustration here. That moment when you realise you are running out of something that holds importance in your life on so many levels.

Meanwhile my best friend Ruia, in Aotearoa New Zealand, was undergoing chemotherapy treatment. The thing consuming her was to survive the game of treatment and life, no matter what. The thing consuming my mind was coffee beans. I was frustrated that I might run out of my favourite coffee beans and she was riding every possible emotion under the sun and going through lifesaving chemotherapy treatment. Her two young children worried that when they woke up in the morning their Mum wouldn't be there to greet them with her usual vigour and enthusiasm. Her husband feared the worst possible outcome, wondering what the hell he and his beautiful wife did to deserve this ridiculous life-changing trauma.

Makes you think, doesn't it. Maybe you are complaining about how tough Covid-19 lockdowns and restrictions are or were. Maybe you are complaining about someone not listening to you, the state of the carpet, the car that needs upgrading, the new shoes you'd love to have. Maybe you are complaining about not receiving funding for a project, someone ignoring you, or someone leaving their dirty laundry on the floor.

There are many things you might be focusing on or complaining about, and in these moments of realisation, we get the opportunity to pause, check-in and revisit our priorities. We get to re-focus on our purpose, our intentions and the meaning beyond ourselves and why we are here.

When we look at someone else's situation, especially when it comes down to life or death situations, it puts things into perspective. Perspective on what we do have, rather than what we don't have. Perspective on who really matters in our lives rather than who doesn't. Perspective on what we believe is truly important rather than things that aren't.

If we allow ourselves to delve into that space of self-awareness and open our eyes to the limitless possibilities in that moment, we gain a new appreciation of others and what they may be experiencing. We gain a fresh perspective on our emotional state and our thoughts. Perspective on what we deem in that current moment to be all-consuming, and the biggest deal in our life. And a fresh perspective on how we are impacting those around us.

This is not about comparison. As Theodore Roosevelt once said, "Comparison is the thief of joy". If we compare ourselves to others, we are looking to either be inferior or superior to them. When we do this comparison, we get caught up in judgemental thoughts of what they have that we don't, how much better they are at something than we are, or who is worse or better off. These judgemental thoughts consume us and disperse any ability to find joy in life.

Comparing one person's situation to another does not serve either individual well and also robs both of the joy in that moment. It is a choice we can make. Whether we go down the rabbit hole of comparison and lose our joy in life, or choose a different perspective and maintain our sense of purpose and meaning beyond ourselves.

Even in times of suffering we have the ability to prioritise and re-focus. As Viktor Frankl identified, suffering can be a meaningful experience, even when facing an incurable illness or the inner dignity of dying. Imagine that for a moment. In the face of death, an individual can still experience the accomplishment of maintaining a chosen attitude, living in an optimistic state, and carrying out their purpose in the best way possible.

I am part of an inspirational group of hard-core mentally tough people (David Goggins Motivational Group), and one particular person Ethan, following a rare brain cancer diagnosis, faced incredible pain, setbacks, surgery, inability to find anything that could numb the pain from five surgeries, wound infections and trauma. He STILL maintained his amazing attitude around this. Right up to his last breath he was inspiring and encouraging others. Within every moment of adversity or trauma that we experience there is a lesson that can be learnt, a message we can receive, or a legacy we can leave in the world, no matter what. The pathway we choose is always our choice.

In that crazed moment of searching for coffee beans, while my best friend was searching for life, I re-adjusted my perspective in line with my meaning and purpose. I became present and thought about what I do have in life, and the many possible options I could take. I laughed at my stupidity and checked in on Ruia to see how she was doing 'today'.

I am pleased to say that since that moment I have a consistent supply of coffee beans, and always remember to check-in on my frustrations. I have also shared many special coffee moments with Ruia on Facetime as we laugh and cry together throughout her journey! She is doing extremely well despite the harsh impact the medication, chemicals, radiation and surgery has had on her body, mind and soul. Her challenging journey continues with ongoing treatment, future surgery and lifelong side effects.

I embrace hope and optimism and know that I will one day soon have the pleasure of sharing a coffee with Ruia and her whanau (family) in person, as soon as the pandemic allows international travel. I also know this. When I live 'on purpose' I share fun and inspiration with everyone around me - my wife, my friends, clients and strangers, anyone I meet in a day. No matter what is happening, I get to choose!

When we consciously choose to make the best of a tough situation and align our thoughts with our purpose, we are able to bring the best version of ourselves to every moment. No matter what. I draw on the lessons from past challenging and demanding situations that have tried and tested me. I revisit (not relive) those moments when I have had to dig deep into my grit and determination. I was a little unsure at first but remember those times when I have overcome and conquered. I instigate my resilient infinite mindset and the belief that I can make it through this moment and the next, and the next, and the next. I know for a fact that Ruia does this too. My amazing wife Elizabeth certainly does.

This technique of delving into past triumphs and times of adversity to recognise our incredible accomplishments, is known as the *Cookie Jar*. The cookie jar concept comes from David Goggins (2018), retired Navy Seal, endurance runner and inspirational person. Goggins has competed in more than sixty ultra-marathons, triathlons and ultra-triathlons, and lives his life with one of the toughest mindsets on the planet. He is regarded as the toughest man alive. He is the only member of the US Armed Forces to complete SEAL training, US Army Ranger School, and Air Force Tactical Air Controller training. His life story epitomises abuse, trauma, racism, heartache and suffering. Yet he found a way to endure and conquer all of it.

The cookie jar is one of the most powerful weapons he personally has. Whenever he is under pressure, be it physical, emotional or mental, he reaches into his metaphorical cookie jar which contains all the things he has overcome, the accomplishments and the traumas, and remembers these with pride. He then uses this moment to push harder, be stronger, and rise even higher! In times of pressure, even the most 'badass' person forgets how strong they are. They get caught up in the sadness, the toughness, the trauma of the moment, and forget how strong and powerful they really are.

Often in moments of adversity we are consumed by the event and unable to find our inner mental, physical and emotional strength or power. This is the moment to reach in and grab a cookie! Goggins' cookie jar contains every single failure and success of his life. When he reaches in and pulls one out, he is reminded of how 'badass' he really is and how he can overcome ANYTHING!

I celebrate my cookie jar in those moments of toughness and stretch when I am not quite sure of what to do next. I am also aware that Ruia is conquering her way through her cancer journey using her metaphorical cookie jar. She revisits the tough stuff and the accomplishments she has got through and reminds herself how 'badass' she is in these times. The ability to dip into those metaphorical cookies, and breathe in the success of getting through a previous situation, is the ultimate reminder of what you have inside and what you can continue to do.

To create your cookie jar, set aside 20 – 30 minutes to start with, and allow yourself to open up, be vulnerable and honest with yourself. Grab a jar (the bigger the better) and some small pieces of paper. Write down (one on each piece) the things that have tested you, the things that have stretched you, and those accomplishments you have dominated. No matter how big or small, recognise them, remember them and celebrate them. You have come through every single one of them, because you are here today, reading this book!

You will be amazed at the number of times you have dug deep, had a courageous conversation, been to hell and back, survived the tough times, turned around a setback, or unleashed your awesomeness in a situation and come out on top. Write down all of those times and place them in your cookie jar.

Sometimes it may feel challenging to revisit the tough times. Remember you only need to revisit, not relive them. These are times you have survived and maybe even thrived in spite of them. Identify all the mental, physical and emotional challenges that you have overpowered. Think about all those times when you thought you couldn't go any further or give more, and then you did. Put those into your cookie jar.

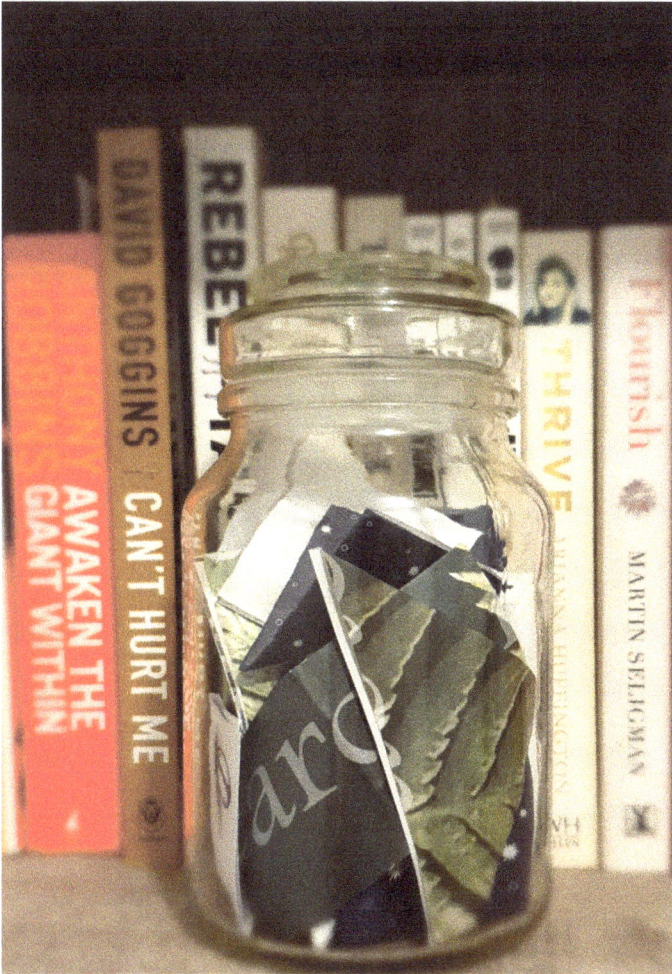

My cookie jar reminds me of all the tough stuff I have experienced, mastered, conquered and overpowered. Some of those moments I have mentioned in this book, and many I have not. It is a reminder of just how 'badass' I am.

For example, enduring both legs in plaster at the same time after Achilles tendon surgery, and then six months later representing New Zealand at Indoor Hockey in Canada. Crashing off my bike and sustaining concussion while biking around Mount Taranaki, New Zealand and getting back up to finish the 150km challenge. Muddling through a redundancy and not finding work for six months.

There are many more moments I have conquered and unleashed my 'badass' powers on. We all have them. Sometimes we just need to delve a little deeper, open up, be vulnerable and discover them. In those times when you need to remember how 'badass' you are, dip your hand in your cookie jar (physical or metaphorical), unleash your GRIT and radiate your ability to bounce forward. It will be one of the most powerful weapons you will ever have. It is in that moment that we realise we are bigger than our circumstances.

Bigger than your circumstances

The crucial element to living your best life with forward momentum and unleashing your most powerful weapon is to have the belief that you are always BIGGER than your Circumstances. ALWAYS! I have more check-ups to go, foods I am still unable to digest, scars, tattoos and muscular challenges. And I can honestly say these challenges only make me stronger – mentally, physically, emotionally and spiritually.

It is not the external world that dictates to me who I BE in life. It is not my circumstances, not the uncontrollable moments, not the check-ups or the thoughtless shallow comments from others, that direct which path I take in life. It is my choice. My choice to go in the direction that serves me well, to follow my purpose with intention and consciousness.

To be the person I am destined to be, to follow my why and find my path. In the words of my wee Scottish 5 foot 2½ inch mother, "there is always a way".

You can either buckle and be destroyed by the enormity of the events that happen in your life or you can draw on all your weapons, face them head on and walk straight into it. Many people spend long periods of their life searching for true happiness, meaningful loving relationships, and a greater sense of their own authentic strengths. It sounds like all of life's psychological wonders wrapped up into a magnificent bundle of bliss. How brilliant it would be if we could experience all of this, with ease and grace! It would be magnificent, right?

However, this is not the case. Being able to bounce forward or experience post traumatic growth comes at a cost. The cost of encountering a traumatic event that rocks you to your core and profoundly affects your purpose in life, and severely alters your sense of meaning. The cost of being in a place of uncertainty where you get to choose. Imagine if you could unleash the most astounding life you could possibly envision. Well, you can. If you choose to.

I now live my life to the fullest. I am fitter, healthier and happier than I have ever been and loving it. I am CEO of our company WALT Institute – Women Authentic Leadership Training Institute and loving it. I am the 'team leader' of an incredible team of people impacting the world. I have an astonishing relationship with my wife that deepens every day.

I have received the most amazing gifts and opportunities. I connect with the most brilliant minds in their fields, and know that there is so much more to come. I can honestly say this is not what I had imagined for myself at any stage of my life. But thank goodness I embraced that life changing moment, faced it head-on with a formidable team around me, and unleashed my weaponry with unspeakable vigour.

My challenge now to you, is to go forth and be awesome. Participate fully in your life with urgency and action to find your purpose, engage your resilience and flourish.

And please remember:

You can **always** be bigger than your circumstances if you remain open to the limitless possibilities that are presenting themselves to you, every single day!

Your limitless possibilities...

1) Live your life with purpose
   - Discover your *why*
   - Align your thinking with your why
2) Maintain perspective on the things that really matter
   - Live your life, not someone elses
   - Allow yourself to step back from the chaos
3) Find meaning in the suffering
   - Notice the lessons to be learned in the tough times
   - Embrace all the opportunities
4) Workout how *badass* you really are
   - Create your cookie jar
   - Fill it with the tough stuff and the accomplishments
5) Choose to live your best life no matter what
6) There is always a way!

EPILOGUE

What's the message from me for you?

My message for you is, live every single day of your life as the best version of you! I am not saying that you must be at 100% every single day. What I mean here is to live each day as the best of who you can BE in that moment. If this is 45% today then you give 45/45% for the day. If you can launch forth into the day at full throttle, giving 100%, then go for it. Remember to pace yourself of course too.

Have fun, be weird, be crazy, learn new things and make massive mistakes along the way. The mistakes are guaranteed anyway and the lessons you can learn from them, to pivot, shift and go again are priceless. It's the only way to do life, if you want to enjoy your life.

If I got to live my earlier years over again, I'd dare to make more mistakes. I'd take more chances, and trust myself more to be okay in those moments when I had no idea what I was doing.

What can change your life? Many things. A moment of deep inspiring thought, a decision you choose to make, or an action you take. I can definitely say, you never know what is around the corner that can impact or change your life in an instant. What I do know is that change is inevitable. It is not to be feared and the only thing I can control is how I respond to it.

This is your key too. You get to choose how you respond to every single situation in your life.

My hope for you is that you live your life with optimism and forward momentum. Live your life knowing that everything happens FOR you, not to you.

Instead of asking why me? Ask, what can I learn from this moment, event, or situation?

Finally, as you come to the end of this book, but not the end of your growth and development, I want to say how much I respect and appreciate you as a person. We may have only met briefly in the pages of this book but it sure feels like we have created a connection, doesn't it? Thank you for allowing me to share my learnings, my teachings and my gift with you. I sincerely hope you implement many of your learnings and new-found strategies so you too can bounce forward and enhance the quality of your life.

I hope we can stay in touch, whether that is through social media, face-to-face at one of our seminars or workshops, or by chance as our paths cross. Please be sure to introduce yourself and I look forward to hearing about your awesomeness.

Remember life is all about the choices we make, no matter what the situation is we are experiencing.

Go forth, be awesome, smile plenty and BE the best version of yourself today and always.

'Life is what you create, so create your best yet.'
– CHRISTINE BURNS –

REFERENCES

American Psychological Association. (2022, June 20). *APA Dictionary of psychology*. https://dictionary.apa.org/

Anglesio, M. S., Papadopoulos, N., Ayhan, A., Nazeran, T. M., Noë, M., Horlings, H. M., Lum, A., Jones, S., Senz, J., Seckin, T., Ho, J., Wu, R. C., Lac, V., Ogawa, H., Tessier-Cloutier, B., Alhassan, R., Wang, A., Wang, Y., Cohen, J. D., Wong, F., … Shih, I. M. (2017). Cancer-Associated Mutations in Endometriosis without Cancer. *The New England journal of medicine*, *376*(19), 1835-1848. https://doi.org/10.1056/NEJMoa1614814

Baumeister, R. F., & Tierney, J. (2012). *Willpower: Rediscovering the greatest human strength*. Penguin.

Bonanno, G. A. (2004). Loss, trauma, and human resilience: have we underestimated the human capacity to thrive after extremely aversive events? *American psychologist*, *59*(1), 20. https://doi.org/10.1037/0003-066X.59.1.20

Brown, B. (2015). *Rising strong*. Random House.

Buettner, D. (2008). The Blue Zones: Lessons for Living Longer from the People Who've Lived the Longest. National Geographic.

Cacioppo, J. T., Gardner, W. L., & Berntson, G. G. (1997). Beyond bipolar conceptualizations and measures: The case of attitudes and evaluative space. *Personality and Social Psychology Review*, *1*(1), 3-25. https://doi.org/10.1207/s15327957pspr0101_2

Carr, C. M. (2006). Sport psychology: psychologic issues and applications.

Physical Medicine and Rehabilitation Clinics, 17(3), 519-535. https://doi.org/10.1016/j.pmr.2006.05.007

Carver, C. S., Scheier, M. F., & Segerstrom, S. C. (2010). Optimism. *Clinical psychology review, 30*(7), 879-889. https://doi.org/10.1016/j.cpr.2010.01.006

Csikszentmihalyi, M. (2011). *Flow: the psychology of optimal experience.* HarperCollins.

Diener, E., & Chan, M. Y. (2011). Happy people live longer: Subjective well-being contributes to health and longevity. *Applied Psychology: Health and Well-Being, 3*(1), 1-43. https://doi.org/10.1111/j.1758-0854.2010.01045.x

Diener, E., Fujita, F., Tay, L., & Biswas-Diener, R. (2012). Purpose, mood, and pleasure in predicting satisfaction judgments. *Social indicators research, 105*(3), 333-341. DOI: 10.1007/s11205-011-9787-8

Duckworth, A. (2016). *Grit: The power of passion and perseverance.* Scribner.

Duckworth, A. L., Peterson, C., Matthews, M. D., & Kelly, D. R. (2007). Grit: perseverance and passion for long-term goals. *Journal of personality and social psychology, 92*(6), 1087. https://doi.org/10.1037/0022-3514.92.6.1087

Dweck, C. (2017). *Mindset-Changing the Way You Think to Fulfil Your Potential.* Robinson.

Emoto, M. (2007). *The Miracle of Water.* Simon and Schuster.

Fredrickson, B. (2013). *Positivity: Groundbreaking research to release your inner optimist and thrive.* Oneworld Publications.

Frankl, V. E. (1992). *Man's search for meaning: An introduction to logotherapy* (4th ed.). Beacon Press.

Gosnell, C. L., & Gable, S. L. (2017). You deplete me: Impacts of providing positive and negative event support on self-control.

Personal Relationships, *24*(3), 598-622. https://doi.org/10.1111/pere.12200

Hassed, C. (2008). *The essence of health: the seven pillars of wellbeing*. Ebury Press.

Hefferon, K., & Boniwell, I. (2011). *Positive Psychology: Theory, research and applications*. McGraw-Hill House.

Hill, N. (1987). *Think and grow rich*. Fawcett Crest.

Horst, K. C., Fero, K. E., Haimovitz, K., & Dweck, C. S. (2012). Abstract P6-08-10: Cancer as self: a novel assessment of patient identity as it relates to a cancer diagnosis. *Cancer Research*, *72*(24_Supplement), P6-08.10. https://doi.org/10.1158/0008-5472.SABCS12-P6-08-10

Ito, T. A., Larsen, J. T., Smith, N. K., & Cacioppo, J. T. (1998). Negative information weighs more heavily on the brain: the negativity bias in evaluative categorizations. *Journal of personality and social psychology*, *75*(4), 887-900. https://doi.org/10.1037/0022-3514.75.4.887

Kashdan, T., & Biswas-Diener, R. (2014). *The upside of your dark side: Why being your whole self–not just your "good" self–drives success and fulfillment*. Penguin.

Kashdan, T. B., & McKnight, P. E. (2009). Origins of purpose in life: Refining our understanding of a life well lived. *Psihologijske teme*, *18*(2), 303-313.

Kiken, L. G., & Fredrickson, B. L. (2017). Cognitive aspects of positive emotions: A broader view for well-being. In Robinson M., Eid M. (eds), *The happy mind: Cognitive contributions to well-being* (pp. 157-175). Springer, Cham. https://doi.org/10.1007/978-3-319-58763-9_9

Korb, A. (2015). *The upward spiral: Using neuroscience to reverse the course of depression, one small change at a time*. New Harbinger Publications.

Langley, S. & Francis, S. (2015, April 20). Harnessing strengths at work. http://www.langleygroup.com.au

Lopez, S. J., & Snyder, C. R. (Eds.). (2009). *The Oxford Handbook of Positive Psychology*. Oxford University Press.

Lyubomirsky, S., Dickerhoof, R., Boehm, J. K., & Sheldon, K. M. (2011). Becoming happier takes both a will and a proper way: an experimental longitudinal intervention to boost well-being. *Emotion*, *11*(2), 391-402. https://doi.org/10.1037/a0022575

Mischel, W., & Ebbesen, E. B. (1970). Attention in delay of gratification. *Journal of personality and social psychology*, *16*(2), 329-337. https://doi.org/10.1037/h0029815

McCrae, R. R., & Costa, P. T. (1987). Validation of the five-factor model of personality across instruments and observers. *Journal of personality and social psychology*, *52*(1), 81-90. https://doi.org/10.1037/0022-3514.52.1.81

McKnight, P. E., & Kashdan, T. B. (2009). Purpose in life as a system that creates and sustains health and well-being: An integrative, testable theory. *Review of general Psychology*, *13*(3), 242-251. https://doi.org/10.1037/a0017152

Oishi, S., & Diener, E. (2014). Residents of poor nations have a greater sense of meaning in life than residents of wealthy nations. *Psychological Science*, *25*(2), 422-430. https://doi.org/10.1177/0956797613507286

Oshio, A., Taku, K., Hirano, M., & Saeed, G. (2018). Resilience and Big Five personality traits: A meta-analysis. *Personality and individual differences*, *127*, 54-60. https://doi.org/10.1016/j.paid.2018.01.048

Rasmussen, H. N., Scheier, M. F., & Greenhouse, J. B. (2009). Optimism and physical health: A meta-analytic review. *Annals of behavioral medicine*, *37*(3), 239-256. https://doi.org/10.1007/s12160-009-9111-x

Rotter, J. B. (1954). General Principles for a Social Learning Framework of Personality Study. In J. B. Rotter, *Social learning and clinical psychology.* (pp. 82-104). Prentice-Hall. https://doi.org/10.1037/10788-004

Rotter, J. B. (1966). Generalized expectancies for internal versus external control of reinforcement. *Psychological Monographs: General and Applied, 80*(1), 1-28. https://doi.org/10.1037/h0092976

Sandberg, S., & Grant, A. (2017). *Option B.* Ebury Publishing.

Segerstrom, S. C. (2005). Optimism and immunity: do positive thoughts always lead to positive effects? *Brain, behavior, and immunity, 19*(3), 195-200. https://doi.org/10.1016/j.bbi.2004.08.003

Segerstrom, S. C., Evans, D. R., & Eisenlohr-Moul, T. A. (2011). Optimism and pessimism dimensions in the Life Orientation Test-Revised: Method and meaning. *Journal of Research in Personality, 45*(1), 126-129. https://doi.org/10.1016/j.jrp.2010.11.007

Seligman, M. E. (2012). *Flourish: A visionary new understanding of happiness and well-being.* Simon and Schuster.

Seligman, M. E., Steen, T. A., Park, N., & Peterson, C. (2005). Positive psychology progress: empirical validation of interventions. *American psychologist, 60*(5), 410-421. https://doi.org/10.1037/0003-066X.60.5.410

Schaefer, S. M., Morozink Boylan, J., Van Reekum, C. M., Lapate, R. C., Norris, C. J., Ryff, C. D., & Davidson, R. J. (2013). Purpose in life predicts better emotional recovery from negative stimuli. *PloS ONE, 8*(11), e80329. https://doi.org/10.1371/journal.pone.0080329

Rashid, Tayyab, & Seligman, Martin. (2019). *Positive Psychotherapy.* Oxford University Press. 10.1093/med-psych/9780195325386.001.0001

Tedeschi, R. G., & Calhoun, L. G. (1996). The Posttraumatic Growth Inventory: Measuring the positive legacy of trauma. *Journal of traumatic stress, 9*(3), 455-471. https://doi.org/10.1007/BF02103658

Tay, L., & Diener, E. (2011). Needs and subjective well-being around the world. *Journal of personality and social psychology, 101*(2), 354. DOI: 10.1037/a0023779

Tedeschi, R. G., & Calhoun, L. G. (2016). Posttraumatic growth. In H. S. Friedman (Ed.), *Encyclopedia of mental health* (2 ed., pp. 305-307). Academic Press.

Tugade, M. M., & Fredrickson, B. L. (2007). Regulation of positive emotions: Emotion regulation strategies that promote resilience. *Journal of happiness studies, 8*(3), 311-333. https://doi.org/10.1007/s10902-006-9015-4

Vaish, A., Grossmann, T., & Woodward, A. (2008). Not all emotions are created equal: the negativity bias in social-emotional development. *Psychological bulletin, 134*(3), 383-403. https://doi.org/10.1037/0033-2909.134.3.383

Vonasch, A. J., Vohs, K. D., Pocheptsova Ghosh, A., & Baumeister, R. F. (2017). Ego depletion induces mental passivity: Behavioral effects beyond impulse control. *Motivation Science, 3*(4), 321-336. https://doi.org/10.1037/mot0000058

Von Culin, K. R., Tsukayama, E., & Duckworth, A. L. (2014). Unpacking grit: Motivational correlates of perseverance and passion for long-term goals. *The Journal of Positive Psychology, 9*(4), 306-312. https://doi.org/10.1080/17439760.2014.898320

AUTHOR BIO

Christine is the Co-founder and CEO of WALT Institute, a global coaching, training and research company empowering people in Science, Technology, Engineering, Math and Medicine (STEMM) to step into their own Authentic Leadership truth.

As a former elite athlete, Christine brings her expertise of coaching and training to both individuals and teams. Typically, she works with professionals, researchers, and academics in Universities, Medical and Science Institutes, and business organisations. Her clients include international dancers, iconic sports teams and individuals, and many high achieving STEMM professionals. She is committed to working with anyone who is ready to take action and unleash their true Authentic self.

ACKNOWLEDGEMENTS

Great things are done by a series of small things brought together.
— Vincent Van Gogh —

This book is a result of a great deal of blood, sweat and tears and so much support from the people who inspired me daily. It started with my amazing wife who encouraged me to share my story with others who are facing adversity, so they know there is a different way to face it and conquer it.

I want to thank Dr Elizabeth Pritchard, my co-writer. One of the best parts of writing this book was going through this journey with you. We shared many tears, laughs, moments, glasses of wine and it was my absolute pleasure to have your wisdom within this book. Thank you for encouraging me to find and share my truth.

Thank you to Susan McLachlan, my incredible editor, for your insights and dedication to help with edits and rewrites, even while you were going through your own adversity. Your brilliant editing and sage advice helped make this book come to life.

Thank you to all the writers, authors, thought leaders and changemakers whose evidence, insights and stories are featured in this book.

To the amazing team I had at Moorabbin Hospital and Peter MacCallum Cancer Centre my deepest gratitude. Thank you for making the dark moments a whole lot brighter and the future look radiantly possible! We made it!

Thank you to so many other people who contributed with time, energy, financial assistance, flowers, food, coffee, wine and good laughs. Thank you for thinking of me and Elizabeth!

www.ingramcontent.com/pod-product-compliance
Lightning Source LLC
Chambersburg PA
CBHW052011030426
42334CB00029BA/3176